"It is refreshing to read a therapy book that is so transparent and generous in detail about what actually goes on in treatment. Steve is a consummate professional, and there is much to be learned from his case studies. His writing is engaging and highly readable, reminiscent of Yalom. I strongly recommend this book for practitioners and patients alike."

Rhena Branch, *author and BABCP accredited practitioner, trainer, and supervisor in the UK. She is director and clinical lead for the mental health charity Fig Branch.*

Working on the Frontline of Mental Health

Working on the Frontline of Mental Health is an account of the day-to-day work in psychological therapies, highlighting not only the complexities clients present but also their remarkable and moving stories of recovery after many years of adversity.

Steve Sheward, a CBT therapist working on the frontline in the NHS and private practice, presents an overview of different psychological presentations, including depression, anxiety, PTSD, OCD, and panic disorder, amongst others. Each chapter provides a detailed description of the latest cognitive-behavioural therapy approaches used to help clients overcome psychological challenges which is paired with compelling case studies that demonstrate their application. The book also outlines the challenges of continuing to deliver therapy during the COVID pandemic, as well as the demands placed upon the profession and the psychological challenges experienced by therapists.

This book will be of interest to a variety of mental health professionals, especially those trained in CBT, along with those who have personal experience of mental health problems and the general reader.

Steve Sheward is a senior CBT and EMDR therapist in the National Health Service and in private practice, where he treats clients presenting with a range of psychological problems, including depression, anxiety, obsessive–compulsive disorder, and post-traumatic stress disorder. He has previously worked as a senior manager within the national careers service.

Working on the Frontline of Mental Health

A CBT Therapist's Casebook

Steve Sheward

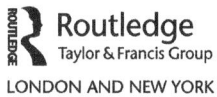
Routledge
Taylor & Francis Group

LONDON AND NEW YORK

Cover image: Getty Images

First published 2023
by Routledge
4 Park Square, Milton Park, Abingdon, Oxon OX14 4RN

and by Routledge
605 Third Avenue, New York, NY 10158

Routledge is an imprint of the Taylor & Francis Group, an informa business

British Library Cataloguing-in-Publication Data
A catalogue record for this book is available from the British Library

Library of Congress Cataloging-in-Publication Data
A catalog record for this book has been requested

ISBN: 978-0-367-55051-6 (hbk)
ISBN: 978-0-367-55050-9 (pbk)
ISBN: 978-1-003-09174-5 (ebk)

DOI: 10.4324/9781003091745

Typeset in Times New Roman
by Apex CoVantage, LLC

This book is dedicated to the memory of my mother,
Elizabeth Sheward

10 October 1923–7 May 2021

Contents

Author's Note

The narratives described in this book are based on my experiences of working as a CBT therapist. I have changed the identifying features of all clients and colleagues who have appeared within this book to protect their privacy. Many elements of the individual case studies have also been merged to protect clients' and colleagues' privacy. Any similarities are purely coincidental.

Introduction

I vividly remember my very first day working as a CBT therapist within the NHS. It was a cold winter morning many years ago when I presented myself at the hospital reception area to the clinical lead of the service who was later to become my supervisor and a source of wisdom and support. I remember being very excited as the prospect of working in the NHS seemed like a big break for me. Prior to this, I had combined working as a therapist in an Adult Education college with running training courses for career advisers since graduating with my MSc in CBT at Goldsmiths College, south London. Therapy was my second career after leaving my job as the Director of the careers service in south London to retrain so I'd given it a lot of consideration, most of it naïve. To be honest, I was influenced by stereotypes in films and TV programmes and envisioned myself sitting in a room surrounded by books and dispensing wisdom to grateful clients. The college therapist role felt like a humble beginning, and I thought that the NHS job would be closer to my fantasy. The reality couldn't have been more different, and when I was confronted with it on my first day, it felt like a punch to the solar plexus.

The morning began amiably enough when the clinical lead took me for a coffee and briefed me on my new role in his office—it happened to be crammed with psychology books from floor to ceiling but then he was the clinical lead and a voracious reader. I frantically made notes on the different structures and procedures described in a jargon that seemed completely alien to me. I was beginning to sense a creeping suspicion that I would be on a steep learning curve. After the briefing, he told me that a patient was due to arrive and we would both be carrying out a clinical assessment. I drew in a breath—this was completely unexpected. I was expecting a gentle induction and didn't realise that my clinical skills (or lack of them) would be scrutinised by the head of service on my first day. I managed a smile that must have seemed like a grimace.

The patient was ushered in and offered a chair and promptly burst into tears before any questions were asked. I watched the clinical lead calm the patient down and carry out a concise assessment within the allotted 50 minutes with an easy expertise that immediately impressed me but increased my feelings of being a rank amateur and imposter. As the patient's sad narrative poured out I was confronted with issues that I hadn't mentally prepared for, including talk of suicidal

DOI: 10.4324/9781003091745-1

ideation. I had been trained in risk management but had only experienced one minor incident when a client had mentioned occasional thoughts that they'd rather not be here but gave firm assurances that they would never do anything to harm themselves. This patient had taken an overdose twice before and was contemplating the same course of action. I was also shocked by the complexity of social and financial challenges that they faced including debt, unemployment, and marital breakdown. I was convinced that I wouldn't have coped with their situation let alone feel confident that I could help solve their problems.

After the session concluded, we had a de-brief and mercifully I wasn't asked too many probing questions. I was given leave to visit the Trust HR department to have my photograph taken and obtain my NHS badge and was invited to return later that afternoon. It was a relief to escape what I perceived to be the oppressive atmosphere of the hospital and travel by public transport to the HR department. But when I arrived at the site, my anxiety started to rise again as I navigated the campus and found the HR department. My feeling of being an imposter was intensified by my surroundings which seemed so *clinical*. Everyone appeared to stride around with an aura of professional purpose and it felt as though I'd penetrated a highly disciplined service that would soon detect my deception and call security.

I managed to present my documents for scrutiny including my qualifications, and they were deemed adequate, much to my relief. A member of the HR team took a mug-shot, and I was duly presented with my NHS badge and lanyard although for quite some time it felt on loan.

I left the campus feeling too nervous to enter the canteen and opted for a seedy transport café near the tube station. By this time I felt so overwhelmed that I called my wife at work and told her that I didn't think I could carry this off—I had worked myself up into a complete lather. She was somewhat sympathetic but pointed out the irony of the situation that I was supposed to be a CBT therapist and was cracking up at the first hurdle. So I took a few deep breaths and tried to obtain a more balanced perspective. On my journey back to the hospital, I reflected on my reaction and concluded that it was my punishment for being complacent. This was a big step-up for me and a big responsibility. I resigned myself to the fact that I would have to work really hard to fill the gaps in my knowledge but isn't that what I wanted—to be the best therapist I could? I went home that evening with the clinical lead's words ringing in my ears: "In this service there is no hiding place—we pride ourself on excellence." I think this was meant to encourage me as to the high standard of the service rather than terrify me.

And so my journey as an NHS CBT therapist began. In spite of my rather terrifying first day, I was given a structured induction into the service and time to familiarise myself with the key clinical protocols before I saw my first patient. At this point, it's important to explain that although CBT might seem like a generic therapeutic approach to those less familiar with it there are various treatment methods, or protocols, recommended by the National Institute of Health and Care Excellence (NICE) based on empirical evidence as to their efficacy. This means that although there may be some general similarities, a CBT protocol for depression will look very different from a protocol for Post-Traumatic Stress Disorder (PTSD), Obsessive Compulsive Disorder (OCD), or other psychological presentations. One way of describing a protocol is as a manualised programme describing step by step and in great detail what the therapist does to support the client throughout treatment. A great deal of emphasis is placed on carrying out treatment whilst closely adhering to the protocol as evidence gathered from clinical trials has indicated that this gives the best chance of a successful outcome for the patient. Clinicians are closely supervised so that they do not "drift" away from the protocol by making their own adaptations although with experience some creativity is helpful within the general framework of the protocol. You will find many examples of clinical protocols in the chapters that follow.

For the first couple of months, I burned the midnight oil reading protocols and was closely supervised each week on my work with patients. I realised that the clinical lead's statement about there being no hiding place in the service wasn't mere hyperbole, and there was and is a high level of scrutiny to ensure client safety and professional standards within primary care mental health services. Typically, a full-time therapist will meet with their clinical supervisor once each week for at least an hour to review client cases and measure progress. As all of the therapy delivered is predicated on evidence-based practice, clients are required to complete validated clinical questionnaires each session and their scores are scrutinised during supervision. As the service has a target of 50% of clients recovering from their presentation, any lack of progress is closely scrutinised in supervision. In addition to quantitative measures, therapists regularly present recordings of their sessions in supervision to maintain quality standards.

Although the work required for my steep learning curve was demanding, it was also stimulating and as I gained confidence, I no longer felt like an imposter and began to inhabit my role. I was also rewarded by being able to take part in outstanding training opportunities and attended workshops with world experts in CBT many delivered in the august environs of the Maudsley Hospital, a centre of excellence in mental health based in south London. I was fortunate in this as I had entered the NHS shortly after the nationwide IAPT service had been launched.

Improving Access to Psychological Therapies (IAPT) was launched in October 2008 and was the brainchild of Richard Layard a labour economist at the London School of Economics and Professor David Clark, a clinical psychologist and lead for the Centre for Anxiety Disorders and Trauma at the Maudsley Hospital. They had both campaigned for a national mental health service with NICE recommended treatments, predominantly CBT and "The Depression Report" (referred to as "the Layard Report") published by the LSE in 2006 put forward the argument for an expanded psychotherapy service within the NHS which eventually facilitated the launch of the IAPT service in 2008. One of the strongest arguments made in the report was that the labour government of the day would see a return on its investment through reductions in benefits as unemployed individuals suffering from depression would be helped to reach recovery and return to work. [1]10 years after the launch of IAPT, the NHS has trained 10,500 therapists and deployed them in the new psychological therapy services and by 2019 the IAPT service has seen over a million people each year.

I am eternally grateful for the many years I spent working within the IAPT service as it has provided me with the knowledge, skills, and confidence to develop my own private CBT practice. The nature of this type of work is equally demanding as the majority of my referrals are from medico-legal firms, but it has also provided me with the opportunity to work with a wide range of complex presentations for longer periods of time than is possible when delivering brief therapy within a primary care setting.

This book is my personal attempt to describe the role of CBT therapists working on the frontline of mental health and to celebrate their compassion and commitment to the profession. In the year that this book was written and published, both clients and therapists rose to the huge challenge that the COVID virus inflicted upon them and I refer to this in the concluding chapter. I hope that the book provides not only an insight into the nature and complexity of the work but also how transformative CBT therapy can be when it works. It's also a testimony to the courage of so many clients who apply themselves to the demands of therapy in spite of the many challenges they face. Perhaps some who read this book will be encouraged to take up the cause and train as a CBT therapist: you are most welcome to join us!

My final ambition for this book is that it will demystify CBT therapy for readers and de-stigmatise the mental health problems described in the following chapters. In doing so, I hope to encourage anyone who thinks they need support to seek professional help rather than suffer in silence. Mental health has become a key issue for the future of humankind—we have to give it parity of esteem with physical health.

Steve Sheward
November 2021

Note

1 IAPT at 10: Achievements and challenges Blog by Professor David M Clark. 13 February 2019

Chapter 1

"What's Happening Now?"

A Journey Into Post-Traumatic Stress Disorder

Ross's Story

When I meet Ross for the first time, I'm immediately struck by the apparent sense of physical menace that he exudes. He looks to be in his late fifties but tall, lean, and muscular. He has many visible tattoos and a broken nose (I later learn that he was a keen amateur boxer). He seems angry with me when I meet him and as we enter the room the atmosphere feels uncomfortable and I'm wondering how we will get along with one another. One of the first tasks of therapy is to create what's referred to as a "strong clinical alliance." This basically means that you need to develop sufficient rapport and trust with a complete stranger so that they will trust you with their most intimate secrets and engage in treatment that is emotionally demanding and very often painful before a cure can be affected. So as Ross and I sit down together, I wonder how to start. He is watching me very closely and I sense that he is taking in every micro-expression on my face and evaluating my body language. We both know why we're here.

Ross has previously completed a course of CBT therapy to stabilise his symptoms of PTSD. He has learnt about his trauma symptoms, why he experiences nightmares and flashbacks, and how therapy will help him to process his traumatic memories. He has also been taught grounding techniques so that if he finds himself dissociating during a flashback or after a nightmare he can pull himself back into the present moment by holding comforting objects or using soothing fragrances: lavender is a popular choice. A very important part of stabilisation focuses on enabling clients to develop an imagined calm place as a mental refuge from their trauma memories. This is particularly important as clients' symptoms frequently worsen during the early stages of therapy as their brains begin the onerous task of processing trauma memories that have been kept at bay through willpower for many years. Clients are encouraged to evoke a pleasant, vivid memory of a time when they felt calm, happy, and safe. They are taught to relive these memories like a virtual reality experience and allow them to unfold moment by

DOI: 10.4324/9781003091745-2

moment whilst paying attention to their five senses. Sadly, many clients suffering from childhood trauma are unable to recall a single memory of feeling safe and we have to use other methods to help them create an imaginary sanctuary. Ross informs me that his calm place is a lake he visited in France when he was 20. So now that Ross has completed all of this preparation during his previous course of therapy, the day has arrived for us to work specifically on his trauma memories.

I begin by checking in with Ross as to how he has been since his last treatment episode and he tells me that nothing's changed, he's still experiencing the same symptoms. This is certainly borne out by the scores on his clinical measures which are within the severe range but fortunately there is no indication that I need to be concerned about his risk status. I start to talk about client confidentiality, and he makes an impatient side-swiping gesture with his large boxer's hand.

"I just want to get on with it."

I can see that it has taken Ross a great deal of determination to attend therapy and confront his trauma memories for the first time in his life and figure that the best thing I can do under the circumstances is to do as he asks me.

I'm going to use imagery rescripting as part of Ross's treatment plan. I'll be following a method devised by an amazing psychologist who I had read avidly and whose workshop I had attended called Arnoud Arntz, professor of Clinical Psychology at the University of Amsterdam. Arntz and his colleagues developed a form of imagery rescripting that follows a specific procedure (Arntz and Weertman, 1999). The client is asked to identify a traumatic childhood memory but is then encouraged to return to the event and observe it happening as their adult self. The final stage of this process is for the client to re-experience the event from the perspective of their young self but with their adult self present.

"What I'd like us to do during this session Ross, is to begin working on one of the memories you've outlined. We'll take it slowly and you're completely in charge. If you want to stop at any point or slow things down I'll follow your lead. How does that sound?" Ross is looking at the floor and he frowns.

"We can start with the one that's kept coming up year after year. Yeah, we might as well start there." By now Ross is gripping his knees and his body is very tense.

"OK Ross. How do you feel about going back to the memory with your eyes closed? Are you comfortable with that or would you prefer to keep your eyes open?" Ross looks at the floor for a few moments and then replies.

"No, it's ok—I'll do it with my eyes shut."

"Good, let's make a start. What I'd like you to do is go back to the memory as though your actually there now aged 6. I need you to tell me what's happening moment by moment exactly as your experiencing it." Ross has closed his eyes and needs no further prompting.

"It's Saturday night and my mum's away visiting her sister in Manchester. I've been left alone with him. We've watched match of the day together and nothing's happened but now I'm lying in bed and it's dark. The house is very quiet." Ross pauses for some time and I resist the temptation to prompt him. He seems to be listening for something, and he inclines his head to the left slightly.

"I can hear a door opening downstairs and there are very light footsteps in the passage. Now I can hear slow footsteps climbing up the stairs. There's a creak and now there's a pause." Ross has begun to perspire heavily and sweat is running down his face.

"The footsteps have reached the top of the stairs and now they're on the landing. I can hear them coming towards my room. The door's opening slowly." Ross is visibly agitated now, and his hands are shaking as they grip his knees. I decide to intervene as I don't want him to become too overwhelmed.

"OK Ross, I want you to leave this place. You're back by the lake in France right now—tell me what you can see."

"I can see oaks and pines all around me. The sunlight's filtering through the leaves onto the lake and it's soft and golden. I can see the sunlight catching on the surface of the water and I can feel it on my face from time to time. There's a very faint breeze and everything is still. The only thing I can hear is birdsong in the distance. I'm breathing in the scent of the pine deeply."

"And how do you feel, standing by the lake?" It's an obvious question but I want to check to see whether Ross's level of distress has decreased sufficiently.

"I feel very calm now." He also looks calm as he has sunken back his chair and is no longer gripping his knees. I am satisfied that Ross has practiced this technique many times and is capable of managing his levels of distress without my support. I need this reassurance before we go any further as there is a distinct possibility that our work on Ross's memories will increase the nightmares and flashbacks he experiences before he is able to fully process his trauma memories. I decide to draw him back into the room.

"That's good. I just want you to focus on that feeling of calm in your body and now gently notice the feeling of the chair your sitting in. Now gradually start to come back into the room and, when you're ready, open your eyes very slowly and bring that feeling of calm with you."

Ross opens his eyes and although he is calm, tears are coursing down his cheeks. He pauses for a while and then begins speaking in an even tone that gradually becomes more agitated.

"It always happened that way. Mum would be away visiting her sister in Manchester and I'd know what was coming. I'd be in bed and hear him coming up the stairs. He'd always open the door slowly and then I'd feel him getting into bed with me in the dark. I can still smell his horrible cheap aftershave and the stink of cigarettes on his breath. He told me that I wasn't to tell anyone, that it was our secret." Whilst I don't want Ross to become too distressed during our first session, I'm also mindful of the fact that this is the first time he has spoken to anyone about the events that he has experienced in childhood and I remain silent whilst he continues.

"I never knew my real dad. Mum told me that he'd left us when I was very young and he didn't keep in touch. So, Vic became a father to me and in spite of everything that he'd done, I cried my eyes out 10 years ago at his funeral after he'd died of cancer—I was heartbroken. Some of the memories I have of him are the happiest and the worst at the same time. I remember the night he took me to Hamley's before Christmas and to see the lights in Oxford Street as a special treat when mum was working as an evening cleaner. He was so kind to me but when we picked up the car on the way back from the station, he made me touch him."

I pass Ross the box of tissues on the table next to us and he wipes his eyes.

"When I grew older, when I boxed, I'd never have a shower with other blokes around. I was always frightened about how I would react. I know it's an odd thing to say, but I often feel as though it was partly my fault. Because, at the time, I didn't mind what he did."

This is a big issue for Ross to disclose, and I can see from his pained expression that it has taken a great deal of courage to share this with me. Tragically many victims of abuse blame themselves for a sexual response in their body that was automatic and beyond their control at the time. Professor Helen Kennerley (2000) has written sensitively about the way the human body is "programmed" to respond to sexual stimulation, in children as well as adults, and that some elements of the abuse experience (e.g. hugs, physical affection) may be pleasurable. I frequently recommend her book, *Overcoming Childhood Trauma* to clients as it helps them clarify this misunderstood response. However, we are nearing the end of our session and I want to make sure that my intervention is timed for maximum effect so I check that Ross is ok and we agree to meet the following week. I ask one last question.

"Well done for today's session Ross, you did brilliantly. I want you to practice calm place imagery and all of the grounding techniques that you've learned throughout the week. If anything comes up that your concerned about, just make a note of it and we can discuss it at our next session. One final thing. Do you think you could find a photo of yourself from when you were aged 6 and bring it along next week?"

Ross agrees without questioning my motive behind the request and as we part company I feel more at ease than when we began the session an hour earlier.

The following week I greet Ross and he is visibly less tense. There is none of the aura of physical menace that I had intuited at our first meeting. I go through our regular procedure of taking the scores from the clinical measures that I use each session. Unsurprisingly, the scores have remained at the high end over the past week. Ross reaches into his pocket and hands me a photo of a shy-looking young boy in a cardigan. He has sad eyes and is looking directly into the camera. Ross explains:

"It was our annual school photograph. I don't know why but they thought it was important for the kids and their parents to have a photo each year. I don't remember when it was taken or what was going on at the time." I thank Ross and ask if he minds me putting the photo to one side on the table next to us and he consents. I ask how he has been over the past week and he responds.

"The nightmares have got worse, I have to say. The wife told me that I've been shouting in my sleep. I've had flashbacks in the day and there's something new."

Ross grimaces and says with disgust:

"There's this feeling . . . down here." He points to his backside. I realise that Ross is experiencing what is described in clinical terms as a somatic flashback. Most people are familiar with the visual and aural elements of re-living trauma experiences, and they are often depicted dramatically in films and plays. One of the lesser-known aspects of PTSD is the way in which physical sensations experienced at the time of the trauma can be stored in the memory and re-experienced if triggered. I remembered a particularly vivid example of this phenomenon described to me by a tutor at a trauma workshop. She described treating a woman suffering from PTSD following an attempt to strangle her. Apparently, red handprints would appear on either side of the woman's neck during therapy sessions when she recalled the incident evoking the shape of the strangler's hands. The Dutch psychiatrist and trauma expert Bessel van der Kolk has written famously about this phenomenon in his book, *The Body Keeps the Score* (van der Kolk, 2014), and I endeavour to explain this reaction to Ross as sensitively as I can and ask him if he is willing to return to the memory we started working on the previous week. He nods silently and I explain the focus of our session.

"I'd like to try something slightly different this time. What I'd like you to do is imagine that you're back in the bedroom as you are now looking in on your 6-year-old self, young Ross. Just let the memory unfold as though it's actually happening moment-by moment but this time you're watching your younger self. Can we try that?" At this point, I don't want to provide too much explanation or direction as I'm hoping that I will be able to work with Ross's spontaneous reactions as he returns to the memory. Ross is visibly apprehensive but he assents silently. He closes his eyes, reclines in the chair, and journeys back to the bedroom of his childhood, a place he has tried to forget all his adult life.

"I'm standing in the bedroom and it's dark but there's some moonlight and I can see myself lying under the covers. I can hear him breathing and I know he's awake. Now I can hear a door opening very softly downstairs and there are light footsteps in the hall. The footsteps are coming up the stairs, very slowly, there's a slight creak halfway up and they're getting closer. I can see little Ross tensing under the bedclothes." I notice that Ross's hands are trembling slightly but he seems to be managing so I let him continue.

"The footsteps are on the upstairs landing now and they're coming towards the bedroom. Now I can see the door handle turning, there's just enough moonlight, and the door is inching open. He's coming into the room, he closes the door quietly and he's standing there looking at little Ross in his bed. He's walking towards the bed." I decide that it's time to intervene and say to Ross:

"What do you want to do?"

"I want to stop him."

"Do it Ross, stop him!"

Ross's whole body tenses and he seems to be shrinking in the chair. He says:

"I can't do it!"

It seems as though this big, powerfully built man is cowering in front of his abuser, rendered helpless. I now have to intervene directly.

"OK Ross, I want you to freeze everything. He can't move—he's just standing there. Have you done that?" Ross nods.

"Now I want you to stand in front of him and tell me what you can see." I am trying to expose Ross to the memory of his abuser in the same way I would expose someone with arachnophobia to a spider. The principle is the same: Ross needs to tolerate the presence of his abuser until his anxiety subsides significantly. He begins tentatively; his eyes seem to have adjusted to the darkness in the bedroom.

"His eyes look cold and glassy . . . his skin is blotchy and I can see the broken veins on his nose. He stinks of cheap aftershave and fags. He's wearing a crumpled blue shirt and a pair of dark slacks. I can see that he's wearing brown slippers."

"How do you feel standing in front of him?"

"I feel disgusted, scared."

"What do you want to do?"

"I want to get him away from here, get him away from little Ross but I can't, he's too much for me." Although I sense that Ross's anxiety has declined somewhat and he is able to tolerate his abuser's presence, it seems as though Ross is not yet able to oppose him. I ask him:

"Is there anyone who could help you and little Ross right now?" He shakes his head slowly; he looks dejected.

"What if I stop him Ross, would that help you both?" He nods and says yes.

"OK, I'm coming through the door and I'm walking up to him. What's he doing?"

"He looks surprised, angry. He's telling you to get out."

"I'm pinning his arm behind his back and I'm dragging him across the room. I'm going to take him away and get him arrested. We're going through the bedroom door, down the stairs and out of the house. What's happening now?"

"Little Ross is sitting up in bed, he looks really scared."

"I want you to do something now. Go towards little Ross. Drop down onto your knees and now look into his eyes—tell me what you can see."

"He looks really sad and alone, his eyes are moist."

"What do you want to do?"

"I want to give him a cuddle." I can see that Ross is crying silently as his arms reach out to embrace little Ross.

"Do you want to ask him what he needs right now?"

"He's telling me that he wants me to take him away from this house. I'm picking him up and carrying him through the bedroom. We're going down the stairs, along the hall and out through the front door. I'm telling him that I'll take him to my home where he'll be safe."

"Is there anything else that he needs?"

"No, he's happy now."

After several moments, Ross gradually opens his eyes and re-adjusts himself to his surroundings in the room. He seems quite calm now and I give him time to regain his composure before asking him about the impressions he had gained from the experience. He answers in a reflective tone of voice.

"He looked so small and vulnerable, little Ross—totally innocent." At this moment I pick up the photograph on the table next to us and hand it to Ross and ask him:

"Do you really think it was this little boy's fault, what happened back then?" Ross looks at the photo and shakes his head. I want to build on this apparent insight and sustain the momentum. I want Ross to go back to the memory again but this time from the perspective of his younger self. In spite of the fact that he was unable to stand up to his abuser, I am confident that he can take care of his younger self after the tenderness he demonstrated. So we return to the dark room where young Ross is lying in bed alone and afraid, listening to the footsteps travelling up the stairs and along the landing.

"I can hear the bedroom door opening with a slight creak and the footsteps have stopped in the room. I'm under the cover and I have my back to him but I know he's looking at me—I can smell his horrible aftershave. I can hear him moving towards the bed."

"Ok. Can you open your eyes and see who else is in the room with you?"

"I can see that you've come into the room with older Ross. Your dragging Vic out of the room and older Ross is hugging me and telling me not to be afraid and that I'm safe now."

"Is there anything that you need from older Ross? Can you ask him?"

"I'm asking him to take me away from here to somewhere safe. He takes me to his home and says that I can stay there. He makes me something to eat and talks to me. I'm getting tired now so I ask him if I can go to bed. He tucks me in and reads me a story. I'm falling asleep now—I feel safe."

Ross falls silent. He is lying back in the chair with his eyes still shut, and it really does seem as though he has fallen asleep. I check my watch and see that we still have some time left and decide to let him savour the peace of this moment. I have witnessed this effect a number of times in therapy when clients experience a deep sense of peace, their younger self cared for in a way that was absent at the time. Eventually, Ross opens his eyes and attunes himself to his surroundings. I check that he is feeling ok and we agree to meet at the same time the following week. I want to avoid an analytical discussion of what has just taken place as Ross has just experienced past events in a profoundly emotional way. It's my hunch that his mind will continue to process the past event and any new insights that he has gained long after he has left the room. As he gets up to leave, he pauses, picks up the small photograph on the desk, and puts it inside his jacket pocket.

Over the following weeks, we revisit other memories from Ross's childhood and on each occasion he experiences them from the perspective of his older self and then his younger self. I observe the emotional bond growing between the two of them and the way in which older Ross is becoming a father to his younger self. Young Ross is experiencing the parental love and warmth he needed at the time untainted by the motives of his stepfather. I also notice how older Ross is becoming increasingly confident in standing up to his stepfather so that my role as protector is no longer required. He is now able to threaten his abuser with the Police as he rescues young Ross. We eventually reach the stage when Ross is ready to work on the final memory, the visit to Hamley's toy store before Christmas. When we first discussed this memory, Ross had expressed a marked ambivalence about the event and described it as one of his best and worse childhood memories. I am curious to see how this rescripting will evolve and avoid asking Ross any questions before we commence as I don't want to influence the direction he will take in any way. We enter the memory from older Ross's perspective.

"I'm in the station car park and there's a blanket of snow covering the ground. It's cold but pleasant because it feels Christmassy and there's a clear sky so the moon has lit everything. The air smells very clean and I also notice that one of the houses nearby must be burning a coal fire. There's no one in the car park. Suddenly Vic's green Ford Anglia is pulling into the car park and I can see little Ross in the passenger seat next to him. Vic is parking at the far end by a thick tree where it's difficult to see the car from the station. I know why he's done that and it's part of his plan for when he and little Ross return from the west end. Vic is getting out of the car and he's walking in the opposite direction to the station. He's left little Ross in the car whilst visiting the tobacconist's kiosk. Before he can get much further across the car park I approach him and he stops in front of me. I say to him, 'You're not taking little Ross to London—you're staying here.' He laughs at me and tells me to piss off. He's about to set off when I throw a right hook that catches him square on his jaw and he goes down into the snow. He's scrabbling around and I kick him in the ribs. He doubles up and I start shouting, 'You're never going near him again you dirty bastard. If you do, I'll kill you. Stay here and don't move.'"

Ross has yelled this sentence with some force, his face contorted with anger. Ross continues.

"I leave Vic laying in the snow, not moving now, and walk towards his car. I gently open the passenger door and tell young Ross that I'm taking him to see the Christmas lights—he looks very happy. I hold his hand and we walk to the station, buy tickets and wait for the train."

As Ross's narrative unfolds, I realise that he wants to describe the whole event in detail. We will not have time enough during the session for him to experience the re-envisioned memory from the perspective of his younger self and I am concerned that we may miss an opportunity. I decide to direct older Ross to switch his perspective to that of little Ross part way through the narrative. I base this decision on the notion that older Ross has been able to stand up to his abuser conclusively and is more than capable of protecting his younger self. I want little Ross to fully appreciate this experience with a loving carer.

"Ok. I want you to be little Ross now. You're with older Ross and you're on the train—what's happening now?"

"We're pulling into Victoria Station and older Ross is taking my hand as we get off the train. It's very busy and I feel a bit overwhelmed with so many people rushing around. I feel slightly scared as we go down into the underground and take the escalator but I also feel excited. When we reach the platform it's really crowded and I can feel the rumble of the train approaching before it bursts out of the tunnel. When it stops we manage to squeeze into the carriage and I'm pressed against coats smelling of smoke and damp weather. We get off at Oxford Street and are surrounded by even more people crowding up the escalator and as we emerge into Regent Street I can see the Christmas lights for the first time in my life and they're amazing. Older Ross crouches down and asked me what I can see and I describe the star shapes suspended high above the cars and the buses and all of the decorations I can see in the shop windows. Soon we are outside Hamleys and I can't believe how big it is. We stand under the red awnings and look at the Christmas scene in the window, smiling snowmen and fir trees. Older Ross asks me what I want for Christmas and we enter the store stunned by the colour and bright lights and so many toys. Soon we find it and I pick up the box containing the action man that I've wanted all year. He buys it for me, gives me a hug and I've never felt happier."

Ross's narrative comes to a halt and he sits in silence for several minutes. I don't make any intervention because I want him to stay with this feeling for as long as possible. When he comes back into the room he looks reflective but doesn't say anything and I don't want to press him even though I'm curious to know what he made of the experience. I ask him if he's ok, he nods and I accompany him as he leaves. I feel confident that he will be able to take care of himself and after he has left I go for a short walk in an attempt to impose some sort of boundary between the experience I have just shared and the next session that I'm about to commence with a different client. On occasions like this, there may not be a great deal of time to process intense emotional experiences and therapists have to discover their own methods for maintaining some sort of equilibrium.

When we meet the following week, it is our final session and our focus is on reflection and the future rather than processing memories from the past. Ross passes me a small package, and I ask him if I can open it. He nods. It's a large white mug.

"THERAPIST—I'm not in it for the INCOME. I'm in it for the OUTCOME.!" I thank Ross and tell him that I definitely agree with the sentiment. It's always nice to receive a gesture of appreciation that you've made a difference in someone's life. I keep all of the cards I've received from clients in view above my desk as an encouragement for when clinical work sometimes falters and I question my ability to do the job adequately.

Ross tells me that the daytime flashbacks have stopped completely, and the one dream he has experienced during the week was visiting Hamleys as a child at Christmastime—with older Ross. He has also taken other major steps on his path to recovery.

"I went back to the station car park for the first time since it happened. It looks very different now, packed with newish looking cars when back then fewer people drove so it could look like a lonely, desolate place. I don't know what I'd expected from going back there but I didn't feel very much, just kept thinking how different it looked. But the other thing that I did this week was to tell my in-laws about it. I've never told anyone else apart from you and my wife. My mum's long gone and she didn't know about it so I thought telling them would be the next best thing."

"And how did it go?"

"The reason I've never told anyone is because I knew that I wouldn't be able to stand it if they pitied me, if I could see it in their eyes and knew what they were thinking. But they were ok with it. They both gave me a hug and told me that I'd done really well considering what had happened to me. It feels like a great weight's been lifted and I thanked my wife for all the support she's given me."

"That's brilliant, you've done fantastically well Ross. I know it's been challenging for you but I hope you can see that all your courage and hard work has paid off." I want Ross to acknowledge that all the gains he has made in therapy are largely due to his efforts and that my role was to facilitate the work.

We settle down to our last task of developing a *Blueprint and relapse prevention plan.* This is an important final component of therapy as it captures all of the insights clients have experienced throughout the course of their treatment ensuring that they aren't lost. It also summarises the various techniques that clients have found helpful and encourages continued practice along with an awareness of any danger signs that indicate relapse and contingency plans for dealing with these symptoms. The final part of the plan summarises what is described as "reclaiming your life goals." A great deal has been written about post-traumatic growth since Lawrence Calhoun and Richard Tedeschi (2013) coined the term describing the way in which individuals often develop increased resilience as the result of dealing with adversity, including processing traumatic memories. Although this focus can be empowering for many clients who have managed to overcome PTSD, it needs to be handled delicately so that the individual doesn't look back over the many years before treatment as wasted. When I ask Ross if he has any plans for the future, his answer is decisive.

"I want to put something back. I've decided that I'm going to volunteer for the Samaritans. There have been times when I've felt so desperate, I couldn't even talk to my wife. They were brilliant. I've often thought about volunteering but I know that I had to sort myself out first."

I congratulate Ross on his decision and am struck by the thought that the bravery he has shown in therapy has led not only to his recovery but also to the benefit that others in need will derive from his compassionate support.

References

Arntz, A. and Weertman, A (1999). Treatment of childhood memories: Theory and practice. *Behaviour Research and Therapy*, 37, pp. 715–740.

Calhoun, L.G. and Tedeschi, R.G. (2013). *Posttraumatic growth in clinical practice*. New York: Routledge.

Kennerley, H. (2000). *Overcoming childhood trauma—a self-help guide using cognitive behavioural techniques*. London: Robinson.

van der Kolk, B. (2014). *The body keeps the score: Mind, brain and body in the transformation of trauma*. London: Penguin.

Chapter 2

Acquainted With the Night

A Journey Into Depression

Throughout my career in the NHS as a CBT therapist and whilst working in private practice, I have always found depression to be the most challenging mental health problem to work with in brief therapy. With anxiety disorders, I find that there is a nervous energy you can work with. Although clients often struggle with the tasks that are required of them in therapy that invariably take them outside of their comfort zone, they are generally motivated to overcome their problems and will often throw themselves into the work with hope. With depression, however, clients are often exhausted, suffer from a sense of hopelessness, and are pessimistic about the likelihood that therapy will help them. As a therapist, you often have to dig deep into your own emotional reserves to avoid getting drawn into the client's sense of hopelessness and to persevere with each setback.

The founder of Cognitive Behavioural Therapy, Arron Beck (1979), described the conditions for depression as part of his cognitive model of emotional disorder in terms of a *negative cognitive triad*. The self: the individual thinks of themselves as no good, useless, inadequate; the world and others: people are cruel and everything is very difficult; the future: things will never get better, there's no escape.

The *Diagnostic and Statistical Manual of Mental Disorders* (*DSM-5*), the bible for psychiatrists, psychologists, and other mental health workers (2013), has very specific diagnostic criteria for a major depressive disorder. Clients have to present with five or more symptoms over the same 2 weeks, and at least one of the symptoms has to be *depressed mood* or *loss of interest or pleasure*. Other symptoms include significant weight loss or weight gain accompanied by a decrease or an increase in appetite; insomnia or hypersomnia (excessive sleepiness throughout the day); agitation or retardation; fatigue or loss of energy; feelings of worthlessness or excessive guilt; poor concentration or indecisiveness; and thoughts of death and suicide.

Dr. Stirling Moorey is a senior lecturer at the Institute of Psychiatry, and I have had the good fortune to attend his workshops. He refers to *the depression mode* when clients describe how their whole person is affected: how they think, feel, behave, and even the way in which their body works. There is a profound sense of life being devoid of pleasure and satisfaction and feelings of helplessness and

DOI: 10.4324/9781003091745-3

hopelessness descend upon the individual so that they often become preoccupied with thoughts about loss, failure, and worthlessness. When a person is in the grip of depression, their thinking bias will inevitably be negative and the proverbial glass will appear half-empty. But the most pernicious effect of the depression mode is that once activated, often through external events such as losing a partner or being made redundant, it triggers a series of vicious cycles that keep the individual trapped in an ever-declining mood state. Moorey has elucidated these cycles in his elegant "Vicious Flower" model (Moorey, 2010).

Depression inclines the individual to constantly engage in *automatic negative thinking* so that situations that would normally be perceived as neutral or even pleasant are regarded with negativity. This extends to interactions with other people leading to falsely negative interpretations of their behaviour or communications. Inevitably, this form of negative thinking lowers the individual's mood and deepens their depression.

Related to this is another mental behaviour that is triggered by the depression mode, namely, *rumination* and *self-attacking*. If something bad has happened to the individual and they suffer from depression, they are less able to move on with their life and more inclined to brood about what happened to them—the job loss or relationship breakdown I quoted earlier as examples. This churning over of past events in the mind, or rumination, is often a misguided attempt to make sense of what happened and is maintained by the belief that if only the person could find the answer as to why things went wrong, they would be able to obtain closure and move on with their life. Given their negative bias, what is more likely to happen is that the individual will engage in bouts of self-recrimination leading to a further deterioration in mood.

Depression invariably gives rise to other negative *moods* and *emotions*. If the individual is suffering from low mood, they will be more susceptible to feelings of guilt, irritability, sadness, and hopelessness. They may also become increasingly depressed about suffering from depression sensing the loss of their former self and fearing that they will never recover.

A typical and understandable behaviour that someone suffering from depression engages in is *withdrawal* and *avoidance*. Unfortunately, acting in this way has the most significant effect on maintaining depression. Feelings of tiredness, hopelessness, and pessimism draw the depressed individual away from activities they used to enjoy or take pride in and also from the company of others. If everything in life seems bleak and even threatening, the greatest temptation is often to escape and hide under the covers in bed all day leading to an ever-declining lethargy cycle and the inevitable realisation that the problems you seek to avoid are still there when you eventually get out of bed.

In addition to avoidance, depression leads people to engage in a range of *unhelpful behaviours,* often misguided attempts to manage low mood by providing short-term relief but that rebound against the person plunging them into deeper depression. Typical examples include using alcohol or recreational drugs, excessive comfort eating, or retail therapy. Less obvious behaviours include prolonged periods of using pornography or gambling to induce a dopamine hit. Self-harm such as cutting the skin is a common attempt to obtain emotional relief often with dangerous consequences.

Every client I have worked with who has suffered from depression has described the profound effect it has had on their *motivation* and *physical symptoms*. As Moorey notes, depression has the effect of shutting down the individual's whole system at a biological level as they experience psychomotor retardation. This manifests itself in constant feelings of tiredness, reduced libido, disturbed sleep, and poor appetite. Weighed down by the burden of these physical symptoms, the sufferer will lack the energy and motivation to do the very things that would possibly lead to an improvement in mood. Worse of all, if they are unaware of the physiological effects of depression, they may be inclined to blame themselves for being "useless and lazy" and increase their deterioration in mood.

Moorey acknowledges that the depression mode and its resultant vicious cycles do not happen in the absence of factors within the patient's personal *environment*, and their work situation, relationships, and home may all be contributory factors. A constant challenge of working within the NHS and sometimes private practice with medico-legal referrals, when treating clients suffering from depression becomes a battle against feelings of hopelessness, is when confronted with a multiplicity of chronic and often tragic life circumstances. It's not uncommon to meet clients presenting with depression who are unemployed single parents living in poor accommodation with anti-social neighbours and who have been sexually abused in childhood, encountered racism, and have experienced recurrent abusive relationships. Add to that a long-term health condition such as chronic pain or endometriosis and I often begin to wonder what possible impact 12–16 sessions of CBT will have on this person given a range of life circumstances that I personally don't think I would be able to cope with and I find myself admiring their courage. Amazingly, it is often possible to make a positive impact in spite of the challenges I've described, and when that happens it feels incredible.

On this particular morning, I'm sitting opposite Robert, a pale shy-looking man in his late forties, who was due to start therapy with me last week but has informed me that he has just been discharged from his borough's Home Treatment Team so I'm feeling a little apprehensive. Just to provide some context, the Home Treatment Team provides crisis interventions for clients who are actively suicidal and they have been supporting Robert after he was admitted to A&E having taken a large overdose of paracetamol. They have now discharged him but I am looking at the results of the clinical questionnaires he has completed before our session and I am concerned about the scores. The PHQ9 is a measure of depressive symptoms, and question 9 asks the respondent to score the following question: "Thoughts that you would be better off dead or of hurting yourself in some way." Robert has given the highest score: 3, indicating that he thinks this nearly every day. Even more concerning is his response to a supplementary question on risk, the Core-10 which poses the question, "Over the last week I made plans to end my life." Robert's score is the highest again: 4—Nearly every day. His overall scores on the questionnaire indicate that he is suffering from severe depression although I can tell this just by looking at him.

Sadly, risk management is often a major part of the therapist's role, and it can be extremely stressful. All of the colleagues I have worked with and the therapists that I supervise have had unnerving experiences when the client they are treating has reported suicidal ideation. In these instances, it is the clinician's responsibility to agree an adequate safety plan with the client which is often straightforward if they are compliant. But on some occasions, the client may give ambiguous responses to questions about their ability to keep themselves safe. No clear indications that they are making imminent plans to take their life that would justify a crisis referral to their Home Treatment Team and additional support but hints that they are "not sure" they will be able to keep themselves safe over the weekend. This can cause therapists to have the occasional sleepless night, myself included.

So I've just met Robert and the first thing we are doing together is working on a safety plan for him—at least it isn't last thing Friday evening.

I'm keen to establish rapport with Robert and would normally attempt to make a strong start so I try to make the best of the situation by telling him that I really want to help him but have to be sure that he can keep himself safe. He nods and I begin with the intension of us working on his safety plan together. I ask him what had triggered his overdose and he tells me, "It's a bit of a long story." I get a strong sense that he wants me to listen to his story and I figure that he will be more amenable to working on the safety plan after I have born witness to his narrative. I encourage him and he begins.

"It all started several years ago when I suffered a heart attack. It came as a complete shock because I was fit all of my life and played tennis. Also, I work as an electrician so I don't sit behind a desk all day. I made more or less a full recovery but felt depressed for the first few months as I thought that I could no longer be physically active anymore. After a while I managed to come to terms with it and I felt better about the condition and started to try and get fit following my doctor's advice but then problems started in my marriage. I began to suffer from erectile dysfunction although my doctor said it was psychological, because to begin with, I was afraid of having another heart attack but then I found out that my wife was having an affair with a friend of mine and I was devastated. He's a builder and he was helping me to do up our home because it was a bit of a wreck when we bought it. I never saw it coming because he and his wife often had dinner with us.

I moved out of our family home and into a small flat so our two girls could stay with their mother. In spite of everything that happened I told my wife that I would forgive her and wanted us to try to patch things up but I told her that she had to agree never to see Clive again. She agreed but told me that she needed a bit of time on her own before she could consider me moving back in. I was so desperate to be with her and the girls that I went along with it. The following week I'd taken the girls out to the cinema and I was due to drop them back after we'd gone for a meal but I decided to go back to our family home and surprise Michelle, ask her if we could all have a pizza delivered and spend time together. But when we got there Clive was with her in spite of the promise that she'd made and we had a terrible argument in front of the girls.

After that night she refused to have anything to do with me and tried to stop me seeing the girls. I spent my first Christmas alone and I felt terrible. I'd spent years working my guts out to buy that house because I wanted to make it a happy place for the family and by and large it was. Then all of a sudden, I've had a heart attack, I'm in my forties and I'm living in pocky little flat away from my kids. But that wasn't the end of it.

Clive left his wife and moved in with Michelle and the girls. This plunged me into an even deeper depression. I had to put the family home on the market with Michelle's agreement because she wanted her share of the equity. When the sale went through it triggered my second episode of depression which has carried on ever since. Just when I thought I'd lost everything Michelle took the girls and moved to Scotland with Clive. That really broke my heart because in spite of everything, I had hoped that we might get back together, somehow, and be together as a family, but now I knew that it would never happen and I hardly see the girls because they live so far away.

About a year later I was feeling really lonely when I met Clive's wife Joanna at the supermarket. We agreed to go for a drink together and she told me that she was devasted after Clive had left, it had been a complete shock for her too. I guess we were both feeling lonely and we started seeing each other but her teenage son really took against me, he was still missing his dad and felt abandoned. In spite of that we developed feelings for one another and I felt terribly confused and it created a deep depression in me. I felt like I hadn't dealt with the separation from Michelle and felt lonely because I was still depressed and thought that Joanna didn't understand. I told her that I couldn't carry on seeing her while I felt so depressed and she broke down and started crying, told me that she loved me. I still walked away from the situation. A couple of months ago my brother died and I was very close to him. Now the only family I have is my old mum and dad and it feels really miserable—we're all still grieving for my brother."

Robert pauses and for the briefest moment an expression of reflectiveness flickers across his face which until now has remained a picture of misery throughout his sad narrative.

"I don't know if the depression has affected the way I viewed the relationship with Joanna. She has offered to get in touch once I have sorted out my depression."

I ponder on Robert's last reflection. It sounds as though he might be future-oriented, which would be an encouraging indication as far as his suicidal risk is concerned and I wonder if I can gently draw us back to the task of completing his safety plan and assessing his level of risk. I also want to validate his experience because as he has been describing it, I've been trying to imagine what it must have been like to experience the accumulation of blows that life has inflicted upon him and just empathising with Robert has given me an overwhelming sense of bleakness and loneliness. I begin tentatively.

"You've been through an incredible amount. I think anyone would be suffering from depression under the same circumstances, myself included. What made you decide to enter therapy?"

"I thought that I owed it to Joanna after what I've put her through—one last chance to see if I could do something about my depression. And if I could, see if it changes the way I feel about her. She suggested CBT and I've looked into it. I've had counselling in the past and I know that no amount of talking is going to fix the problems I've got."

"Can I ask you, the overdose you took a fortnight ago, what triggered it?"

Robert looks down at the floor and pauses for a moment.

"I'd found out that Michelle and Clive were taking the girls on holiday for the first time—they were all going away together like a proper family. I spoke to both of the girls before they set off and they were both really happy. It was such a blow. It felt as though they'd moved on and didn't need me anymore. I made a big mistake and opened a bottle of scotch that I had in the flat. I polished off most of the bottle and I got really maudlin. When I took the pills, part of the reason was to show them how much pain they'd caused me. I passed out and dad found me. His got a set of keys to my flat and he became worried when I didn't answer my phone. He called an ambulance and I got blue-lighted to A&E."

Suddenly Robert starts to sob convulsively; his whole body wracked with the misery he is feeling.

"I feel so ashamed, putting him through that after my brother died."

I offer Robert water and tissues; eventually, he calms down and agrees to work on a safety plan with me. He is less resistant than I anticipated and I was relieved to find that he was not making active plans to end his life in spite of what he had written on the questionnaire. He did, however, think that he would be better off dead and the main protective factor stopping him from taking his life would be the grief it would cause his mother and father. Sadly, thinking about his daughters would not prevent him from taking his life as he now believed they didn't need him. Robert's thoughts about Joanna offered some vague motivation for suspending plans to end his life and to try to overcome his depression in therapy but he was not optimistic about this outcome. It was for him the "last throw of the dice" and he thought that if anything happened to his mother or father, it would precipitate a more determined attempt.

"I've got it worked out. There's a place on the Kent coast near Dover. I used to go there with mum and dad on holiday when I was a kid—I used to take Michelle and the girls there too. One of my favourite places on the coast is by St Margaret's

Bay. There's a bench there with amazing views over the cliffs and the channel. That's where I'll do it. I won't jump, I'll take sleeping pills and scotch and I'll just slip away watching that view."

I know the area Robert is talking about and have often walked along the same coastal paths with my wife. A few years ago we were walking along one of my favourite stretches of coastline between Ramsgate and Pegwell Bay. At one point you walk through a tree-lined park resounding with birdsong and turn out onto a panoramic view of the sea in the distance. It was a particularly beautiful late spring day and the sea looked almost Mediterranean-blue in the bright sunshine. Along the path, there are a few Victorian rain shelters that had recently been restored, and I noticed that the first one had been partially cordoned off with tape so that passers-by had to avoid the area on the pathway nearest the clifftop. As we approached I noticed that a young policeman was standing in front of the tape. He smiled at me and my wife and gestured down towards the bottom of the cliff and said,

"I doesn't take much figuring out"

The circumstances seemed slightly odd, and I should have realised what had happened before I looked down to the pavement by the sea at the bottom of the cliff where the policeman had gestured. And then I saw the unmistakable shape of a body under a blanket with a leg protruding from it revealing a trainer and denim-clad calf. I felt immensely sad and thought to myself, if only that person had managed to get through the night, they could have been enjoying this beautiful spring day that might have lifted their spirits. But it was a naïve thought because the suicidal are guided by a different logic when their final act is an attempt to seek relief from seemingly interminable suffering or the escape from insurmountable problems.

Fortunately, Robert is reasonably compliant when we begin constructing his safety plan and he agrees to give therapy a chance. We identify risk factors including further indications that his daughters are getting closer to their new "stepdad" and drifting away from him (possibly negative distorted thinking) and identify contingency plans for dealing with his drop in mood other than downing a bottle of scotch. Robert tells me that he is lucky enough to have a close friend, Chris, who cares about him even though Robert feels a burden to him. Chris has urged Robert to call him day or night following his overdose if the urge should take him again. We agree that this will form an important part of Robert's safety plan as well as carrying a photo of his mother and father to remind him of the pain his death would cause them.

The next thing I turn my attention to is Robert's disclosure that he has declined anti-depressant medication although it has been suggested by his GP. I gently probe him about this.

"I really don't want to go down that route. My grandad had psychosis and the medication they put him on turned him into a complete zombie. We used to visit him at the Bethlem and he never came out again."

It's clear that Robert's childhood experiences of bearing witness to his grandfather's decline have given rise to a deep-routed aversion to psycho-tropic medication. I gently explain that what he is suffering from, although severe in its own way, is not as long-standing and debilitating as psychosis and also that medication prescribed for mental health problems these days has evolved significantly since the 1960s. I am concerned that because Robert's symptoms of depression are so severe, he will not be able to engage in the CBT treatment plan I have in mind unless he experiences some elevation in mood and that the quickest way for him to make progress would be a course of anti-depressant medication prescribed by his GP, typically an SSRI or to give the drug its proper name, a selective serotonin reuptake inhibitor. Instead of selling Robert the idea, I explore what he knows about medication and fill the gaps in his knowledge. I explain the role of Serotonin as a neurotransmitter in regulating mood and that SSRIs are thought to prevent the synapses from re-absorbing (or "reuptaking") it so that its lingering presence can improve symptoms of depression and enable clients to respond to treatments like CBT (NHS, 2021). Robert is intrigued by this explanation and, encouragingly, asks me questions.

"But won't I become addicted like my grandfather?"

I explain that antidepressants are not deemed to be addictive but would need to be taken under the supervision of his GP (Camden Primary Care Trust, 2009). I explain that the plan would be for Robert to build up his serotonin levels so that he has sufficient energy and motivation to engage in therapy. I reinforce this point.

"As you know from your own research into CBT, we'll be working together to ensure that you have the skills to overcome depression and prevent any relapse. My goal is to help you to become your own therapist and make myself redundant. Once you've got the skills my hope is that you'll be able to come off medication gradually."

I add that this isn't just my opinion; it's the NICE recommended treatment for depression (NICE, 2009). I pose one further question for Robert.

"Just think about it over the next week. Pharmaceutical companies spend bil-lions of dollars developing medication and carrying out thousands of trials to measure its effectiveness and safety. How does that compare to drinking whisky as a mood enhancer?"

Robert promised to give the issue his serious consideration and revisit the topic at our next session. Before we part company I print off Robert's safety plan and provide him with a copy. I have one last task for him over the com-ing week, and I really need commitment at a time when his motivation is at a low ebb. I provide Robert with a simple diary and ask him to record hour-by-hour what he is doing and thinking. He looks at me askance: how can this mundane piece of admin be in any way connected to relieving him of his suffering? This is one of the challenging initial tasks in CBT therapy when treating depression, and I make every effort to present a compelling argument for completing the task when the client's resources are often at an all-time low.

"I know this seems like a lot to ask of you but it's vitally important that we both gain an understanding of what triggers your low mood and what keeps it going. It's equally important that we find out what lifts your mood. Depression is different for everyone and there are probably patterns of thoughts and behaviours that impact on your mood that you're not even aware of. I just need you to write down briefly what's happening hour-by-hour and what you're thinking at that time. I also need you to rate your mood during the hour in terms of how depressed you feel 0 being no depression at all and 10 representing the most depressed you've felt in your life."

"Ok, I'm willing to go along with it. But why do I have to do it hour-by-hour? I have to work most days and it'll be difficult to keep pulling out a diary and writing down how I'm feeling. Also, I don't want people to see me doing it—they'll think I'm weird. Can't I just do it at the end of the day?"

"I know it's a lot to ask of you but it's really important that you do it hour-by-hour. Let's say you had a reasonable day at work, maybe even had a laugh. Then you got home and had a phone call from your ex-wife, got into an argument. What would that do for your mood?"

"I'd feel shit."

"And when it came to writing about what happened during the day when you're in a bad mood, are you more or less likely to notice the things that made you feel better?"

"Less likely. Ok, I'll do my very best."

"That's great. Now my biggest fear is that come next week when we meet again you'll turn up and won't have completed the diary. Can we think of anything that might get in the way of you completing it hour-by-hour?"

My clinical supervisor has taught me to hammer home this rather dramatic emphasis because it underlines the importance of the task for the client and gives the therapist permission to show dismay at the next session if the diary is not completed—without being punitive ("That was my biggest fear. I'm really sorry, I obviously didn't get across how important the task is. Let me try again."). As things stand, Robert is able to think of a number of potential problems that may prevent him from completing the diary each hour (e.g. working in a customer's home) and we manage to come up with solutions (e.g. complete the diary in the loo).

When Robert returns the following week, I am encouraged by the fact that he has completed the diary reasonably well in spite of his initial reticence. He has also met with his GP and commenced taking a course of 50 mls Sertraline. The GP has informed him that he will not feel the effects of the medication for 4–6 weeks, but it is an encouraging start. We review Robert's diary together starting with Monday's events, and I ask him if he has noticed any patterns regarding the

Day: Monday			Date		
Time	Activity/Thoughts	Mood	Time	Activity	Mood
1–5 am	Lying in bed unable to sleep. Thinking that my life is over, I'll never be happy	9	3 pm	Working but couple of the blokes larking around singing—found it funny	5
6 am	I know it's nearly time to get up but I stay in bed exhausted thinking about how lousy the day will be	9	4 pm	Getting to the end of the day feeling a bit tired	6
7 am	Have a shower	7	5 pm	Drove home with the radio on	5
8 am	Travel to work in the van—still thinking about not seeing the girls this weekend	8	6 pm	Got home and had tea. Felt low because it reminded me that I'm living on my own in some crappy little flat in my forties	7
9 am	Working on a new—build with the blokes—busy	5	7 pm	Watched TV	7
10 am	Working—busy	4/5	8 pm	Watched TV	7
11 am	Tea break. They go off to the café. I stay behind and check my phone. Text from Michelle asking for money for girls' school uniforms—pissed off	8	9 pm	Saw an advert on the TV with a happy looking family in a nice house having a meal together. Reminded me of what I've lost	8/9
12 pm	Back to work	7	10 pm	Changed channels on the TV	8
1 pm	Lunch—sit outside, eat my sandwiches, and look at my phone	8	11 pm	Had a wash. Went to bed. Staring at the ceiling thinking	8/9
2 pm	Back to work	7	12 am	Still can't sleep	8/9

Figure 2.1 Robert's Activity Diary

activities, his thoughts, and their resulting impact on his mood. He looks dejected and replies in a flat, monotone voice.

"My main hang-up is losing the girls and the family home. And why Michelle left me for Clive—how they could both betray me like that. I keep thinking about it to try and find some sort of answer but I can't seem to find a way forward. I'm so disappointed in myself and I just can't let it go, I've just totally messed up everything. I can't seem to break the cycle and getting home every day is a reminder that I'm stuck in a rented bedsit at my age with nothing to show for it."

"I can see that you spend a lot of time thinking about it in bed and it seems to be affecting your sleep."

"My sleep's chronic, I'm completely knackered all of the time. Some nights it gets so bad that I get up and wander over to a common near my flat. There are wild horses and ponies there. I order hay online and feed them sometimes. It helps me forget for just a few moments and calm down a bit."

"I notice that your scores are quite high when you're watching TV: what do you make of that?"

"I don't know. I feel down the moment I get back to the flat because of what it reminds me of and then I feel guilty because I'm not doing enough for mum and dad. They've lost their only other son and I'm a complete failure—they can't see their grandkids anymore. So I try to block it all out by watching TV."

"And how's that working for you?"

"Looking at the diary I can see that it isn't. My mind's constantly wandering and I can't concentrate on what I'm watching."

"And looking at Monday's entries there seems to be another downside to watching TV for you."

"Yeah. . . . All those programmes and adverts with happy families. I hadn't really thought about it before but that can definitely tip me into a really bad mood."

"What about the lower scores—what do you make of what's going on there?"

"From what I can see, they're few and far between but it's usually when something takes my mind away from the constant thinking that's torturing me."

"Like when?"

"When I go to the tools at work I have to concentrate. It's probably the only time I'm not going over things in my mind."

"I also noticed that there was a difference in your mood at work when you were with your mates and when you were deliberately on your own."

"I know. I didn't want to go to the café with them because they'd think I was depressing to be around so I stayed by myself and got that text from Michelle."

"But you seemed to cheer up in the afternoon when they were mucking about a bit."

"It's funny, sometimes it's possible to forget myself even now if they draw me in. But I don't go out with them anymore after work because, as I said, they'd probably find me miserable company."

As we go through the remainder of Robert's diary, it becomes apparent that his patterns of thoughts and behaviours correspond closely with Moorey's vicious cycles that we explored earlier, particularly his constant *rumination* about the loss of the family home and separation from his daughters. And Robert's main way of trying to cope with his symptoms of low mood is remarkably similar to that of most of the clients I have treated for depression—watching TV for hours on end in an attempt to distract themselves from their thoughts and feelings. This is an incredibly unhelpful strategy as it invariably leads to rumination and a return to the very thoughts they seek to escape because, if you are depressed, it is particularly difficult to sustain concentration for more than the briefest of intervals. And at a more subtle level that most people are unaware of, watching TV content can inflict unexpected triggers on the unwary viewer as in Robert's case when he is presented with images of a happy family together—the very thing he has lost. Other triggers can include idyllic romantic relationships as an affront to the lonely and dramas depicting death and loss to torment the bereaved.

It's also apparent from his diary that Robert has withdrawn himself from the company of others largely due to a misguided belief that they don't want to be around him in spite of constant invitations from concerned friends and also from Joanna, who apparently still cares for Robert even after he walked away from the relationship. Robert also disclosed that he has abstained from a number of more active pursuits since he became depressed. In spite of his heart attack, Robert was advised by his GP that he could still play football, go running and visit the gym as long as he built up his stamina gradually and he pursued these activities until his mood and, in particular, his motivation deteriorated. I ponder on this as I map out each of Moorey's vicious cycles on the whiteboard drawing on examples from Roberts' diary. Then I ask him if he has any ideas on how to break out of the cycles. He shakes his head and tells me that if he could figure that out he wouldn't be here so I make an observation to see how he will react and where it will lead us.

"It seems to me as though you've been trying to *think* your way out of your problems—would you say that's a fair comment?"

"Yes, I think that's spot on but I'm not getting anywhere, it's just worse."

"In some ways that's one of the big problems with depression, the more you try to think your way out of it, the more tangled up in your thoughts you get and the worse your mood becomes. Have you ever got stuck in the snow while driving in the winter?"

"Yes, a couple of years ago."

"What happens if you get stuck in a rut and keep your foot on the accelerator?"

"The wheel keeps spinning and you go deeper into the hole. I get that but what am I supposed to do?"

It is at this point that I introduce Robert to the principles of *Behavioural Activation* for depression or BA for short, a psychological therapy for depression with one of the largest evidence bases to demonstrate its effectiveness (Dimidjian et al., 2011 and Ekers et al., 2014). This CBT protocol has been devised by Christopher R Martell and his colleagues (Martell, Dimidjian and Herman-Dunn, 2010), a Clinical Associate Professor at the University of Washington.

Many people assume that psychological therapies involve clients talking about their problems until they obtain some sort of insight or relief—and little else. In fact, there is a significant *behavioural* component in many talking therapies, and it is particularly important when treating depression. As we have seen in Robert's case, thinking his way out of depression isn't working for him and if we continue to talk about his problems each week, although he may derive some temporary relief ("getting things off his chest"), this approach will not lead to an ongoing improvement in his mood and at worst, the sessions may turn into "verbal rumination" which could cause his mood to deteriorate by constantly going over his problems. The emphasis on Behavioural Activation as the name suggests is on getting clients to change how they feel by changing what they do or, to quote the title of Kathryn Bottonari's clinical paper on the subject, *Stop Thinking and Start Doing* (Bottonari, 2008). As we shall see, clients are taught strategies to reduce rumination or *thinking* about their problems and many of the activities they are encouraged to engage in are calculated to give them respite from their thoughts as well as a mood lift through physical exercise and the company of others.

I provide Robert with a simplified explanation of BA and he looks slightly baffled.

"But I can't just bury my head in the sand, these problems aren't going to go away."

"I know that but at the moment your energy levels are on the floor. It's my job to help you improve your mood, motivation and stamina through the work we're going to do together. If we can achieve that, you'll be in a much better state to tackle the challenges you're facing and we can then go into the problem solving phase of the programme. But right now, you need a mental holiday from all that thinking and that's what we have to work on."

I produce a blank diary for the following week, and Robert looks dismayed. I explain to him that the function of the diary is now twofold: to schedule activities that will hopefully improve his mood *and to measure their positive effect;* and to continue to monitor his mood throughout the week so that we can refine our approach.

We discuss which activities Robert could resume that previously improved his mood and he reluctantly agrees to go for a light jog three times each week immediately after he gets home from work and to meet his friend Chris on two evenings for a couple of pints but no excessive drinking. He also agrees to visiting the café for lunch and tea breaks with his workmates rather than moping about on his own.

When we meet the following week, Robert presents his diary which he has partially completed. He reasons that some of the activities are repetitive, but I encourage him to resume his more diligent recording as he may miss subtle details that will help us spot patterns contributing to his shifts in mood, negative or positive. When we review the diary together he concedes that going for a jog three times each week and meeting Chris in the pub had elevated his mood (the depression scores during these periods were low compared with the previous week—three on one occasion) but he makes the point that these moments represent temporary relief. After an hour or two of respite, he descends into a darkened mood preoccupied with the loss of his home and family. Although Robert hasn't filled the diary in with as much detail as I would have preferred, there is sufficient information to indicate that when he plummets into low mood, Robert frequently engages in typical *unhelpful behaviours* that Moorey had described in his series of vicious cycles. I decide that this is a good launching point to introduce Robert to the BA model of TRAP and TRAC (Martell, Dimidjian and Herman-Dunn, 2010).

TRAP is a helpful acronym as it describes accurately the unhelpful behavioural and psychological traps that clients fall into when they are depressed and find it difficult to break out of. One of the recurrent themes of depression is the way in which an individual's actions are frequently dictated by their moods—they respond to situations in often unhelpful ways because of how they are feeling at the time. A typical example of this is planning to get up at a reasonable hour but when the alarm goes, noticing it's a cold and rainy day, feeling immediately gloomy, hiding under the covers, and escaping back into sleep. The aim of teaching clients the TRAP and TRAC model is to help them to stop letting their negative emotions dictate their actions in a reactive way.

I provide Robert with a brief overview and ask him if he would be interested in learning more about this. He seems genuinely curious, possibly because he feels relief at focusing on something more interesting than his diary, and I begin to explain the model by obtaining examples from him and jotting them on the whiteboard.

TRAPs

Trigger: A situation that has an impact on the individual's mood.

Response: A reaction to the trigger, typically a negative emotion.

Avoidance Pattern: The avoidance behaviour, which usually takes the form of an attempt to escape the unpleasant feelings associated with the person's emotional reaction, but one that has unhelpful consequences (e.g. getting drunk to numb the emotional pain after a row with one's partner but waking up later with a hangover).

Triggers vary but usually fall within the following categories:

Historical: Reminders of losses such as the anniversaries of unhappy events. Associations with past events such as sad songs suddenly played on the radio even fragrances that might remind the person of someone they have lost.

Current: Challenging events happening in the here and now like making a difficult phone call or receiving a bill through the post.

External: All of the previous examples are external events—they happen outside of us and trigger an emotional reaction.

Internal: These are more subtle triggers because they happen inside of us and we may not always be aware of them. They often involve our thinking processes such as ruminating and worrying and sometimes dreams can have a powerful emotional impact.

Interpersonal: This is a very specific trigger involving challenging interactions with other people such as difficult conversations and arguments.

Response:

Responses to triggers are often emotional, and in the context of depression they tend to involve negative emotions and attempts to avoid the bad feelings or:

Avoidance patterns:

Examples include procrastination: putting things off to avoid anxiety or boredom.

Thinking angry thoughts about other people who have annoyed you rather than asserting yourself or being passive and taking the blame unduly.

Rumination: constantly brooding about past events, losses, and failures.

Numbing or zoning out by watching hours of TV, getting drunk, or taking drugs.

As mentioned, the depressed individual's attempts to avoid negative emotions may work in the short term, if at all, but usually cause other problems the greatest one being an increased tendency to "bury one's head in the sand" and avoid dealing with life's challenges leading to an increased sense of helplessness and hopelessness.

The main endeavour of this approach is to enable the client to develop *alternative coping strategies* to replace their patterns of avoidance so that they are able to tackle challenges and achieve goals without letting negative emotions dictate their behaviour hence:

TRACs

Trigger
Response
Alternative
Coping

Working through Robert's diary and using this method, we are able to analyse a number of his TRAPs and work out suitable alternative coping strategies or TRACs:

Trigger: Dreaming about losing the home and waking up in the middle night
Response: sadness and guilt

Avoidance Pattern: Ruminating and worrying for 3 hours
Alternative Coping: Get out of bed, go into a different room, and read until feeling tired

Trigger: In the pub with friends and they start talking about mortgages
Response: Sadness, regret

Avoidance Pattern: Zone out; go into myself

Alternative Coping: Force myself to become involved in the conversation; change the subject

Trigger: returning home to my bedsit flat after work
Response: Sadness as it reminds me that I have lost my home

Avoidance Pattern: Sleeping during the day (resulting in poor sleep at night)

Alternative Coping: Go running immediately after returning home or go for a brisk walk

I suggest that we integrate these responses into Robert's weekly routine but he is sceptical: his mood and motivation have been poor for months. How can he magically force himself to break out of these patterns of behaviour? As ever in these situations, I force myself to sound enthusiastic and upbeat even though I am feeling tired.

"Try to think of it like this. You weren't aware of these patterns of behaviour, your personal TRAPs, until today. Now that you're aware of them, you can plan for them. For example, you know that when you return home to your flat the likelihood is that you'll feel low and your usual response will be to brood or take a nap. You can't let that happen—you have to force yourself to go for a run without thinking about it further."

"What if it's raining—what if I don't *feel* like it?"

"One of the most important principles of Behavioural Activation is *act according to a plan, not a mood,* like the Nike advertising slogan, "Just Do It." You saw from your diary that when you take action, when you break this vicious cycle, you feel better. That's the key to climbing out of this hole you've fallen into and getting your life back. And you can help yourself to get motivated."

"How?"

"Make sure you have your running gear ready so that when you get back, you get changed and just go. Don't even think about it. Also, do you like music."

"Yeah, sometimes."

"Ok, music has a huge impact on our moods. I want you to compile a top 20 motivational hits list and play a couple of them when you're driving home from work in the car. Hopefully it'll get you in the mood for a run and stop you from ruminating. Also, do you like movies? Can you think of any films that pump you up?"

Robert is looking at me with a curious expression on his face as I've probably become a bit manic in my attempts to enthuse him but he nods thoughtfully.

"I like the Rocky films, particularly that bit where he runs up the hill and starts dancing about."

"Great idea—brilliant. I want you to find as many Rocky clips on U-tube as you can and play one of them on your mobile just before you get home."

Robert smiles faintly for the first time in our work together and seems amused by my suggestions but I'm hoping that they will have some positive impact on strengthening his motivation. Every hour in which his mood is elevated will count as a small victory in helping him to combat his depression.

When we meet at our next session, Robert presents his diary and reports that he has experienced a rather mixed week of ups and downs. To his credit he has stuck to his scheduled activities and made an effort to work against his TRAPs by utilising the alternative coping strategies that we had devised and this is reflected in improved scores with regard to his depression ratings. But on Sunday's entry, I see that he has scored a 9 after spending the afternoon with his daughters during a rare visit to their aunt in Croydon and he confirms that the aftermath following their visit to London Zoo was his lowest point in the week.

"It just felt as though they didn't want to be there and they couldn't wait to get back home to Scotland."

To compound matters, Robert has fallen into a classic TRAP of trying to drown his sorrows in alcohol after returning to his lonely flat and plummeting into a spiral of rumination about the past, self-recrimination, and depression. This has caused a setback to the positive progress he was making and he has been brooding about his major preoccupation: loss of his family and home. His clinical questionnaire indicates that he has been thinking that he would be better off dead for most days during the week, but thankfully he is not making any plans to take his life. We review Robert's risk plan and I derive some encouragement from the fact that looking at a photo of his mother and father enabled him to disengage from thoughts about taking his life even though he had drunk half a bottle of whisky. I feel despondent for a moment but force myself to focus on Robert's positive achievements and I give him praise for this although he looks crestfallen. I try a different approach.

"Ok, you've had a setback and that's very common when you're battling to overcome depression. From now on we need to plan for similar setbacks like these so that you'll have a strategy in your back pocket to help you get through the situation. But the most important thing is that we learn from what happened so that we can improve our strategy together."

As we analyse what took place Sunday afternoon, it soon becomes apparent that Robert was expecting the girls to be distant towards him. When I gently question him about what evidence he had for them not wanting to be with him, he is unable to provide anything other than a felt sense that they were bored and wanted the trip to the zoo to end.

"Do you think it's possible that because you were expecting them not to want to be with you, that you were seeing things through a negative filter on their behaviour? That you might have read negative signs in their behaviour?"

"I suppose it's possible. I just feel really awkward when I'm with them after everything that's happened."

"Do you think that they might pick up on that? Children are very intuitive and they can tune into body language and the way we say things."

"You're probably right. Next time I'm determined to make a real effort and not let my mood ruin the outing."

"That's great. What else can you learn from what happened afterwards?"

"I suppose, don't drink half a bottle of scotch."

"The outing with the girls was one thing but afterwards you really caused your mood to plummet by brooding about it."

And at this point, I decide that we need to make a huge effort to address Robert's *Rumination,* another one of Sterling Moorey's vicious cycles.

Rumination is an incredibly unhelpful mental behaviour when you are suffering from depression. The word derives from the 16th-century Latin verb *ruminare,* to chew the cud—as cows do (Collins, 1998). The word has evolved as a psychological term to describe unhelpful thought processes including delving into bad things that have happened in the past and going over them repeatedly much in the same way that Robert is doing with regard to his loss of home and family. It also involves obsessing, overthinking, and churning over problems repeatedly without making headway. Some psychologists include worry within this category although rumination normally focuses the mind on past events rather than concern about what might happen in the future although the behaviours are very similar and if you suffer from depression, you may find yourself drifting backwards and forwards between bad things that have happened in the past and even worse things that *might* happen in the future. The emotional consequences of rumination are to plunge us into an increasingly bleak and anxious state of mind which, as we've seen from Stirling Moorey's vicious cycle, feeds our depression. If it's so unhelpful, why do we engage in it?

Addis and Martell (2004) make an interesting observation that in the early 1980s self-help books and the media encouraged people suffering from psychological problems to focus on their "inner child." This meant delving into negative childhood experiences to resolve problems that occur later in life. This approach may be appropriate in different types of therapy (e.g. psychodynamic and schema therapy), but if someone is so depressed they find it challenging to get out of bed and complete routine tasks, this type of deep thinking is thought to be unhelpful in overcoming depression (Nolen-Hoeksema, Parker and Larson, 1994). It's always possible to explore the past for insights at a later stage once the black cloud of depression has dissipated; but as we will see with Robert, being in the present rather than the past, is the best place for him to be at the moment.

The other reason that rumination is such a seductive behaviour is that we are tricked by our brains into believing that if we constantly mull over a negative past event we will be able to find the answer to why it happened and move on, as with Robert's failed marriage, but this rarely happens. We just get stuck in the same negative thought cycles that increase our depression. Part of the problem with worry and rumination is that we are thought to have evolved to think in this way as our ancient ancestors survived because they constantly focused on past losses and future threats to learn from the former and prepare for the latter (Gilbert, 2009). But unless these thought processes lead to constructive action, they just feed our low mood and anxiety needlessly.

As I explain all this to Robert, he recognises the behaviour I'm describing immediately and is genuinely interested in the concepts surrounding it. But he feels helpless in the face of its power over him describing it as an automatic process that takes over against his will. I ask him to describe what he feels and thinks when the process is triggered.

We talk about a recent incident he had identified when he was having a drink in a pub with friends and one of them mentioned the subject of his mortgage.

"The moment he started talking about that my mind jumped to a time when Michelle and I were renewing our mortgage on the house. We were sitting in the garden looking at different repayment packages, just a normal boring task, but I remember it being a lovely sunny day and we were both in a good mood. I was looking around the garden at the kids playing thinking how well we'd done and as I started thinking about that, I felt overwhelming sadness because I knew that I'd never get that back again. It was as though one moment I was in the pub having a laugh, and the next moment I wasn't there at all—my body was there, sitting in the chair but the real me was back in the past."

"That sounds really difficult—does this sort of thing happen often?"

"Yes, it's as though I might be doing something but then I'm distracted by a thought about the past and I'm dragged back there. Sometimes I totally zone out and I might be in my head for an hour or even more if it happens when I'm watching telly."

"And what do you notice about your mood when this happens?"

"I feel really down, it's a heavy feeling."

"Where do you feel it in your body?"

"Usually around my heart like a heavy sadness but my brain becomes really foggy."

"From what you're saying, it sounds as though you *are* able to recognise when this happens."

"I suppose so, it just happens very quickly."

"What if I could help you to recognise the very first signs that you were about to drift into rumination and helped you to learn a strategy to combat it?"

Robert is understandably sceptical about his ability to do this but over the course of the following week I get him to monitor his rumination and pay particular attention to common situations when it's likely to occur, what the content of the rumination is, and what the consequences are in terms of his mood and behaviour. I emphasise that this is an immensely important piece of work and that he needs to become an expert in recognising the subtlest cues that he is about to drift into a bout of rumination.

When we review Robert's findings the following week, it is apparent that he is more likely to ruminate when he has nothing to focus his attention on and he is at his most vulnerable when lying in bed unable to sleep and when watching TV as we had previously discerned from his TRAPs. He also has a tendency to ruminate whilst driving, and this has led to a couple of near misses when he has nearly crashed into the back of the car in front. Returning to his empty flat remains a major trigger but I am encouraged to find that the task of monitoring his rumination has sensitised Robert to the subtle cues that he wasn't previously aware of and he now concedes that the behaviour seems less like an automatic response to internal and external triggers—he believes that he can slow things down and actually interrupt the process. This provides me with an opportunity to introduce the next important component in Robert's treatment and a fundamental BA technique: *Rumination Cues Action—or RCA.*

The essence of *rumination cues action* is to help the client to anticipate typical situations when they are in danger of succumbing, recognise the thoughts and feelings that indicate the first stages of rumination, and take radical action to pull themselves back into the present moment. This is vitally important, and the psychologist Mihaly Csikszentmihalyi (2002) eloquently described the inherent fragility of the human mind and its tendency to vacillate between rumination and worry. He stated that unless we train our minds in some way, without some focus, our thoughts will be drawn to something disturbing, problematic, or painful from the past or future. He describes this as *entropy*—the default state of human consciousness. His remedy is to engage in activities which completely absorb us and focus our attention on the present moment. He describes these experiences as *flow* states, and he uses the testimonies of motorcyclists, ballerinas, sculptors, and even assembly line workers to illustrate this concept. You may have come across a similar description used in sports psychology of athletes being in "the zone" when they are fully absorbed in their performance. Although this may sound rather grandiose when it comes to everyday activities and overcoming depression, the principle is similar: the essence of *rumination cues action* is to use our five senses to ground ourselves in the present moment and stop us from drifting into entropy.

We work on Robert's *actions* that will pull him back into the present moment and give him a "mental holiday" from rumination and worry building on the strategies that he has already begun to practice including listening to music and focusing his attention back on the conversation, getting out of bed, and listening to podcasts when he is unable to sleep. Towards the end of our session, we have managed to compile a checklist of action that Robert will immediately default to at the earliest indication that he may drift into rumination but I also introduce a caveat.

"You may find it challenging at first but this is such an important technique that I want you to really persevere with it. You'll probably find that your mind will wander and you will drift into rumination in spite of your best intentions. But every time you notice that happening and pull yourself back into the present moment, you'll be strengthening neural pathways so that your brain will become less reactive to the triggers that cause you to ruminate and worry. Think of it in the same way to doing reps in the gym to strengthen a particular muscle."

The explanation seems to resonate with Robert as he has commenced going to the gym one day each week as part of his behavioural activation programme. Before we part company he has some news for me.

"I meant to tell you, Joanna got in touch with me and was asking how therapy was going. I told her about some of the things we'd covered and she seemed genuinely interested."

"How did you feel about that?"

"It made me happy, that she was thinking about me—that she hadn't given up on me."

"I've got an idea, can I run it by you?"

"Sure."

"Very often I find it helpful to involve the partners of people I'm working with in their treatment programme. It can help with motivation if someone else is there between therapy sessions to provide encouragement with the assignments. I know you're both not officially "together", but I wondered if you and Joanna would be willing to try out what I've just described. After all, she wanted you to enter therapy and she's interested in your progress."

Robert smiles at this suggestion, and there's a warmth in his expression that gives me cause for optimism.

When we next meet and review Robert's progress, he seems to be doing well at combating rumination and is filling his diary with many more activities during the week than when we first started working together. He is now running and going to the gym three times per week, socialising with friends during the weekend (previously his lowest point was when he spent it alone). He plans to resume playing tennis the coming Sunday. His scores have improved markedly, and it seems that the combination of RCA and increased activities are paying off because he has less time to ruminate and uses these tools to resist this tendency when he notices it creeping in.

On this occasion, I take Robert for a walk through a fountain garden in a small park nearby as the weather is favourable and I want to add to his repertoire of techniques that will help ground himself in the present moment. I ask Robert to turn his attention to what he can see and he describes the marble work of the fountain and surrounding plants, the way the sunlight plays on the water. I then get him to pay attention to what he can hear, and he notices the lilting strains of Classic FM drifting through the open French doors of the adjacent café. It's a rather gentile setting, and it exudes a calming presence as well as a meeting place for many senior citizens who meet on days like these over tea and scones whilst enjoying the sunshine—I look on in envy and fantasise about retirement. Then, I draw Robert's attention to what he can feel and he walks to the bushes growing in a flowerbed nearby. He runs his hands over the leaves and describes their texture and pays attention to the warmth of the sun on his face and a slight breeze. Finally, I ask him if he notices any fragrances and he breaks one of the leaves, inhales its scent, and nods.

"How do you feel now compared with when we started the session."

"Really calm. Even a little bit happy."

I encourage him to practice this method of bringing his attention back to the present moment when he goes walking but caution him not to become frustrated when he notices his mind wandering—just to gently draw his focus back to what he can see, hear, etc. Without me prompting him, Robert sheepishly discloses that Joanna has visited him at his flat and of all things, given him a haircut. It sounds like a warm, intimate act given that he had previously ended their relationship.

"She's really interested in what I'm doing and has come up with more ideas for me around Rumination Cues Action. She's read all of the handouts you gave me too."

"That's really good—I'm pleased."

Robert pauses and I get the sense that there's something important he wants to share with me but is hesitating. I don't say anything because I might risk losing the moment. Eventually, as we go back to the room he confides in me.

"I went for a drink with Chris the evening after Joanna came round and I told him how things had gone. He reckons that he could get us back together if I really wanted it to happen, even with things as they stand."

"And is that what you want?"

"I think so. Chris and his wife Julie are going out with a Joanna and I for a meal. It was their idea and I'm amazed she agreed to it."

We part company and I think of Robert over the weekend hoping that his night out with Joanna goes well. I have a rather simplistic desire for a happy ending and reflect sentimentally that if only they could get back together again, his problems would be solved and his depression alleviated. But that would be too much to hope for and I have to keep my focus on helping Robert to manage his moods more effectively no matter what life throws at him. Nevertheless, when I meet Robert next, I am impatient to hear how his encounter with Joanna had gone.

"Joanna and I went out for dinner with Chris and Julie and it went fine. Strangely it didn't feel as awkward as expected. I saw her by herself a couple of nights ago, we went for a drink together. I told her that I hadn't recognised the olive branch she'd offered me after I said that I couldn't see her anymore because I was so depressed at the time—I just couldn't see beyond the mood I was in. I told her that I wanted to try again, that I really wanted to make it work but she's not sure because she was hurt by my rejection, particularly after Clive leaving her, it would be a big risk if she took me back and it didn't work out. There's also the difficulties with her son accepting me and we'd both have to be patient with him. She asked me if I really meant what I said because I never seemed positive about the relationship in the past. I started crying and told her that I really did. I gave her a hug and I really felt something for her."

Robert is sobbing now and I hand him some tissues. He continues.

"The thing is, I feel so guilty towards everyone because I screwed everything up. If it hadn't been for me we would have been in a much better financial position and I wouldn't have Joanna doubting me because I hurt her."

As I wait for Robert to compose himself, I am thinking rapidly. It seems that he has a slender opportunity to reach out for the things that matter so much to him: a loving partner, a family, and a home. His position seems tenuous because his sense of self-recrimination may cause him to sabotage any chance he has of reclaiming his life and his constant feelings of guilt seem to be the sticking point. After he has calmed down and is able to focus on what I am saying I explore with him the difference between guilt and remorse (Dryden, 2005). He has not come across this distinction before and starts to pay attention as I delineate the differences between the two emotional states. After a while, I notice that our session is coming to an end and attempted a summary.

"So the main difference is that feeling guilt assumes you can never make up for what you've done, you're a thoroughly bad person and you deserve to be punished—that really doesn't seem to be the case with you. Remorse on the other hand, means that you may have done something that you regret but it doesn't make you a bad person and there were mitigating factors in your situation. More importantly, remorse means that you can atone for what you've done—you can put things right without continuing to punish yourself. The big question is, which path to you want to choose now?"

Robert nods slowly and asks if I can email him a description of the two emotions as he wants to reflect on this.

Over the next two sessions, we move on to the final part of Martell's pro-gramme which is very apposite given recent developments, namely, *building the life you want*. Robert has been seeing Joanna two or three times each week, and he tells me that he feels more love for her than when they first got together and fortunately this is reciprocated. He attributes this to the fact that, now that his depressive symptoms have decreased, he is able to view the relationship with more clarity and he is no longer convinced that his desire to be with Joanna is due to a rebound effect following his separation from Michelle and Clive's betrayal of his friendship.

The day comes around when we reach our final session together and we com-plete Robert's Blueprint—a summary of all he has learned in therapy and a relapse prevention plan. Although he has not reached 50% recovery on the clinical meas-ures for depression and anxiety, he has made significant progress and his risk scores are zero.

Robert has a present for me—it's a toy nodding bulldog. He smiles at my reaction.

"Churchill's black dog. We'll I couldn't find a black dog but maybe it's more appropriate for recovery."

It is in fact the Churchillian insurance company mascot that is featured on TV advertising campaigns and has a cheerful expression and white and light brown fur. I thank him for his thoughtful gift and ask how things stand with Joanna.

"It's positive. We're still taking it slowly because she wants to be sure that our relationship is strong before she tells her family. We need to plan things carefully in terms of when and how we tell Michelle, Clive and the girls because we don't know how they will react. Although things are still awkward with her son, there seems to be a bit of a thaw in his coldness towards me. And she thinks that one day I could move in with her so I'm hopeful."

We agree a time and date when I will call Robert to check that he is still manag-ing to keep his depression at bay or if he needs further support. We shake hands and part company.

Three months later, I am poised to make the follow-up phone call with some trepidation. I punch Robert's number into my mobile and listen to the ring tone which eventually goes through to his voice mail. I leave a message reminding him that I am checking in at our arranged time and ask him to call me back if he needs further support. A week goes by and I don't receive an answer. I had hoped to hear that everything had worked out between them—the happy ending that I'd craved—but reflect on the fact that it's part of my work to take leave of clients without knowing where their lives will take them. Although their story has preoccupied me I realise that I have to let it go. I'd like to think that they found home and hearth together and that Robert never thinks of that bench by St. Margaret's Bay along the seafront with the stunning views of the channel.

References

Addis, M.E. and Martell, C.R. (2004). *Overcoming depression one step at a time. The new behavioral approach to getting your life back.* Canada: New Harbinger Publications.

American Psychiatric Association. (2013). Diagnostic and statistical manual of mental disorders, 5th ed. Washington: American Psychiatric Publishing.

Beck, A.T., Rush, A.J., Shaw, B.F. and Emery, G. (1979). *Cognitive therapy of depression.* New York: Guilford Press.

Bottonari, K. (2008). Stop thinking and start doing: Switching from cognitive therapy to behavioral activation in a case of chronic treatment-resistant depression. *Cognitive and Behavioral Practice.* doi: 10.1016/j.cbpra.2008.02.005

Camden Primary Care Trust. (2009). *Antidepressants: Your self-help guide.* London: Copywrite Camden Primary Care Trust.

Collins. (1998). *Collins English dictionary millennium edition.* Glasgow: Harper Collins Publications.

Csikszentmihalyi, M. (2002). *Flow: The psychology of optimal experience.* London: Harper Perennial.

Dimidjian, S., Barrera Jr, M., Martell, C., Munoz, R.F. and Lewinsohn, P.M. (2011). The origins and current status of behavioral activation treatments for depression. *Annual Review of Clinical Psychology,* 7, pp. 1–38.

Dryden, W. (2005). *Fundamentals of rational emotive behaviour therapy.* London: Whurr Publishers Ltd.

Ekers, D., Webster, L., Van Straten, A., Cuijpers, P., Richards, D. and Gilbody, S. (2014). Behavioural activation for depression; An update of meta-analysis of effectiveness and sub group analysis. *PloS One,* 9(6), e100100.

Gilbert, P. (2009). *Overcoming depression. A self-help guide using cognitive behavioral techniques.* London: Constable & Robinson Ltd.

Martell, C.R., Dimidjian, S. and Herman-Dunn, R. (2010). *Behavioral activation for depression.* New York: The Guilford Press.

Moorey, S. (2010). The six cycles maintenance model: Growing a "vicious flower" for depression. *Behavioural and Cognitive Psychotherapy,* 38, pp. 173–184.

NHS. (2021). Overview—Selective serotonin reuptake inhibitors (SSRIs) at www.nhs.uk

NICE. (2009). *1.2 The stepped care model in depression in adults: Recognition and management.* Clinical Guideline (CG90), published: 28 October 2009, London: NICE.

Nolen-Hoeksema, S., Parker, L.E. and Larson, J. (1994). Ruminative coping with depressed mood following loss. *Journal of Personality and Social Psychology,* 677(1), pp. 92–104.

Chapter 3

Feel the Fear

Working With the Generally Anxious

It is our second session, and Gerard and I are reviewing his worry diary. I had asked him to complete this after our first session in order to get an idea of the type of worry he engages in and also to get him into the habit of keeping a worry diary so that he becomes aware of the fact that it is a mental *behaviour* that he engages in and that he can disengage with the process if he chooses to although we have a lot of work to do before he will be able to even consider this as a possibility. When I set other clients this task, they usually provide me with one or two sides of A4 detailing their worries during the week. Gerard has presented me with 10 pages of highly detailed notes, typed rather than handwritten, and neatly presented: he clearly has a lot of worries and definitely meets *DSM-5 criteria for Generalised Anxiety Disorder or GAD as it's commonly known.

Gerard worries excessively and feels anxious for most of his waking life and has done so since early childhood. He tells me that he was an only child and both his parents were worriers. His father suffered from ill health and was frequently unemployed which caused the family to experience ongoing financial insecurity. His propensity to worry increased in secondary school when he was bullied by a group of boys in his year group. He got into the habit of praying that nothing bad would happen to him when he left the house in the morning even though he wasn't religious. Whenever he experienced a "good" day at school and wasn't picked on, he attributed this to his morning prayer. When I ask him if he still engages in this behaviour, he shakes his head and looks slightly embarrassed and I suspect that we will have to return to this issue.

He tells me that it's impossible for him to control his worry and that it ranges arbitrarily as he dwells on potential catastrophes concerning his wife's health (she's very fit apparently), the possibility of redundancy (Gerard and his wife have secure jobs), and of being an inadequate father. He worries a great deal about his job which involves compiling data reports on youth service provision and works late most days due to excessively checking his work. This also involves checking even the most mundane email at least three times before sending it.

Gerard's health is a major source of worry. He has a morbid fear of being diagnosed with testicular cancer and frequently seeks reassurance from his GP. He

DOI: 10.4324/9781003091745-4

knows that researching the illness fuels his anxiety but he struggles to resist the urge as he sits in front of a computer all day at work and the temptation is ever-present. His research isn't confined to the internet and he visits forums and Facebook groups related to cancer. This worry has inflicted not only psychological pain on Gerard but also physical discomfort as he has got into the habit of physically checking his testicles for lumps (the clinical term is "palpating") resulting in soreness that triggers further worry. He also maintains a negative belief that his worrying will make him "go insane" and is constantly scanning himself for sensations of brain fog and gaps in memory as evidence that he is "losing the plot" rather than an understandable consequence of his anxiety.

But Gerard's most distressing worry concerns his 2-year-old daughter, Clara. He does not feel ready to disclose the nature of his worry at this stage and I am wondering if Gerard fears that talking about his greatest fear will make it come true—that would certainly fit with his presentation.

GAD is a pernicious complaint as most clients who are diagnosed with the condition report a poor quality of life as they spend most of their time living in a miserable fear-ridden future rather than in the present moment (Dugas and Robichaud, 2007). Even on holiday in a beautiful setting whilst watching an incredible sunset, the GAD client will only be physically present but unable to focus on the sunset before them. In their minds' eye, they are back at work confronted with the tasks that have accumulated in their absence. Even during their most intimate moments, their mind draws them away from the experience to future concerns. We all worry—it's part of the human condition. But people with GAD are particularly sensitive to *uncertainty* in the way that hay fever sufferers are sensitive to pollen. As my starting point, I want to help Gerard understand the nature of worry rather than getting bogged down in his 10 pages of neatly typed notes although I will return to them afterwards once he is able to differentiate between the different *types* of worry he is engaging in. I know that Gerard has read some CBT self-help books on stress and worry but this hasn't reduced his symptoms. I review what he has learned from his reading, and he diligently recalls basic CBT principles on the relationship between thoughts, emotions, and their influence on behaviour. I continue with a question.

"Why do you think we human beings worry? You know that already, *everybody* worries—but why?"

"Something to do with evolution? I guess it's because it helps us foresee danger."

I ask Gerard if he would be interested in exploring this topic in a little more detail, and he shows genuine interest. I want to gauge how useful spending valuable time on psychoeducation will be. I have to be careful because I find the topic fascinating and need to guard against self-indulgence. Some people find theoretical explanations engrossing and gain insights that motivate them to fully engage in treatment. Others find these discussions abstract, slightly boring and are impatient to learn techniques to intervene in their problem. I'm getting a sense that

Gerard falls into the first group. I begin at the beginning, what the historian Yuval Noah Harari (2014) describes as the *cognitive revolution*, when we became *homo sapiens* approximately 70,000 years ago and developed the ability to use language and our conscious thought emerged as a consequence.

Through whatever arbitrary evolutionary process that occurred, when we developed the *prefrontal cortex,* we developed the ability to use not only language but also mentally time travel and plan (Siegel, 2013). We could envisage and anticipate future dangers, wild animals, or other tribes that might attack us at a certain clearing in the forest, and either avoid the risk or take measures to protect ourselves. We could also use this ability to travel backwards in time to reflect on bad things that had happened to us, eating poisoned berries that made us sick for a week, the insect that stung us on a certain type of plant whilst foraging.

I go to the whiteboard and sketch out a very rudimentary image drawing on my minimal artistic skills:

Natural selection ensured that we have inherited this tendency to focus on negative things that have happened in the past and negative things that *might* happen in the future. Nature doesn't care about our happiness because she's developed a perfect neural mechanism for ensuring our survival and it's hardwired into our brains. The psychologist Mihaly Csikszentmihalyi (pronounced "cheeks sent me high") describes this as one of the unfortunate burdens of

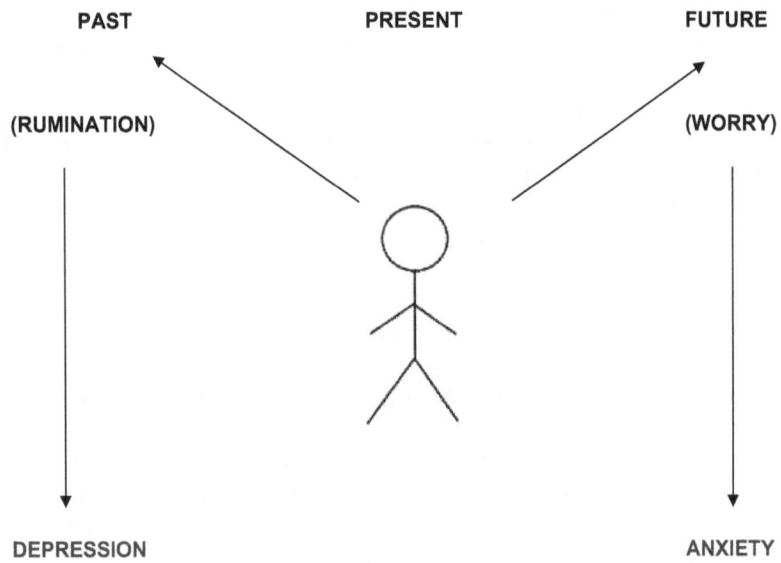

Figure 3.1 Focus of Attention Diagram

human consciousness that the normal state of the mind is *chaos* or *entropy* (Csikszentmihalyi, 2002). He goes further in claiming that, unless we develop the ability to focus our attention adequately, we will be at the whim of our neural hardwiring causing our minds to flit backwards and forwards between rumination and worry subjecting us to waves of anxiety and low mood. You could say that the devil makes work for idle minds. Gerard points to my sketch on the whiteboard.

"I can identify with the process on the right hand side. I seldom spend time going over the past—I'm too busy worrying. So if evolution has given us this response to help us survive, why do I feel so awful all of the time? It can't be good for us."

"What are you concerned about with regards to your worrying?"

"That I'll make myself ill in some way. I even wonder if it could make me vulnerable to cancer." I make a mental note of Gerard's *negative belief about worry* as part of the formulation of his problem that I'm mentally piecing together as we speak. I try to address his question succinctly.

"Worry in and of itself is pretty harmless. It's a mental *behaviour* we carry out in our minds. What you're describing is the emotional consequence of worry, namely *anxiety*. You experience that physically because of the release of the stress hormone cortisol in your brain and adrenaline in your body."

"Is that a fight or flight response?"

"That would be an extreme example if you thought you were in some sort of grave danger. But the amygdala, the fear centre of your brain, is still getting activated at a lower level whenever you worry so your body experiences a constant drip-feed of cortisol and adrenaline. But the good news is that if worry is a thought process rather than an emotion, we can learn ways of detaching from it." Gerard doesn't look convinced so I decided to come back to this point at a later stage and focus on his lengthy worry diary.

"I'd like us to look at your notes and have a think about different types of *triggers* for worry that you're engaged in. We can split these into two categories: external and internal triggers. Can you pull out any examples from your diary?"

"Well, on Monday I got a call from my boss telling me that he needed the report I was working on sooner than expected. I suppose that's an external trigger?"

"Yes, good example. And I see that on a scale of zero to ten for the level of anxiety you experienced, you scored this one as eight so it must have been quite intense. What about an internal trigger?"

"Following on from the phone call, I felt a tightness in my chest and started thinking that I might have a problem with my heart. And then I started thinking."

Gerard becomes tearful at this point and I pause, hand him a tissue, and wait for him to calm down. I'm wondering whether we've touched on the worry that he doesn't feel ready to disclose. After a few moments, he takes a deep breath and asks me to go on. I strive for a gentler tone of voice concerned that I'm sounding too matter of fact.

"That's a really good example of an internal trigger: a physical sensation that caused you to worry about your health. But a worry itself can also be an internal trigger and activate subsequent worries developing into what we call "worry chains": one worry after another going on and on. Does that happen to you?" Gerard nods looking a little more composed.

"Now I really want to emphasize this next bit because it's very important. Based on years of research by leading experts there are basically two types of worry. The first type of worry related to current problems that actually exist; the second type relates what we call *hypothetical* problems that may never happen. Can you point out any examples of *current* problems in your diary?" Gerard scans the pages and alights on an example.

"There's something wrong with the car. The engine keeps juddering when its idling."

"That's spot-on. Now can you show me an example of a worry about a hypothetical problem? The easiest way to identify this type of worry is if it begins with the statement 'what if'."

"It follows on from the previous example, what if I take the car to the garage and it's a huge job—and we can't afford it?"

"So, out of the two problems, which one do you have some control over?"

"The first one."

"Exactly. With current problems, even though they're anxiety provoking, you can come up with a plan to deal with them. How long have you had this problem?"

"Weeks."

"What's stopped you from taking your car to a garage to have it checked out?"

"I'm really worried about what they will say."

Gerard's answer reveals two common challenges that GAD sufferers are faced with. First, avoidance or procrastination as it's often referred to. Gerard avoids the emotional discomfort of increased anxiety that a trip to the garage will cause him but maintains the problem as the car engine's judder is a constant reminder and source of concern. The second challenge he has is around active problem-solving. Research indicates that GAD sufferers are just as capable as anyone else of problem-solving (Dugas and Robichaud, 2007). The difference is that they have a *negative problem orientation* which means that they see problems as threats rather than an inevitable part of life. GAD sufferers don't trust their ability to solve problems and fear that their attempts to resolve the situation will turn out badly. I pick another example from Gerard's diary.

"You've written that on Tuesday evening your wife was late home from work and hadn't called you. You worried that she might have been attacked?"

"Christine's a social worker and sometimes she has to visit clients in areas where there's a lot of criminal activity."

"Has she ever been attacked?"

"No, but it constantly plays on my mind."

"So what type of worry do you think it is?"

"Hypothetical obviously, but it's a real possibility."

"I don't disagree but looking at your diary it seems that most of your worries are hypothetical and may never happen. And the scores are very high. How does it feel when you worry like this?"

"Awful. I feel tense all of the time, my stomach is constantly churning and I suffer from headaches."

"That seems a high price to pay for worrying about events that may and probably will never happen." My last statement was rather crass and I'm punished for my sloppiness by Gerard's frustrated response.

"I know these things may never happen—*but I just can't help worrying like this.*" He shouts the last part of the sentence, apologises, and looks down at the floor. I also apologies for what must have seemed a flippant remark trivialising the years of misery that constant worrying causes and the despondency and exhaustion that Gerard is currently experiencing. I have to tread carefully as he may be pessimistic about my ability to help him.

I ask Gerard to continue with his diary for the next week but this time note what he is worried about three times each day at pre-set times and distinguish between actual and hypothetical worries. Getting him to become aware of this distinction is an essential first step before I can teach Gerard the relevant strategies for dealing with both types of worry. I am also hoping that the very act of noticing his thought processes and standing back from them will enable Gerard to gradually recognise that his anxious thoughts don't have to define him and he can develop the ability to step outside the worry chains that have tormented him for years. The term for this process in psychology is *metacognition,* and it encapsulates a profound insight into the human condition: we are the only animals on the planet that have the ability *to think about our thoughts.* Much of the work in CBT involves mundane tasks like completing thought diaries and analysing the content of the thoughts in a similar way to the task I have encouraged Gerard to engage in. But the laborious task of writing down our thoughts forces us to detach from the[1] 50,000 cognitions we experience *each day* and can help us to obtain an objective perspective on their content. James Joyce famously described this *stream of consciousness* in his 1922 novel *Ulysses* narrating his hero Leopold Bloom's thoughts, feelings, and perceptions as they flowed in often arbitrary tides merging and breaking moment by moment whilst walking the streets of Dublin. Sometimes that stream of consciousness can lead us to creative insights; on other occasions, it can bear us away into darker territories and we'd be better advised to stand on the banks and watch the currents flow by. There's also a neurological rational for taking note of our thoughts and I encourage clients to *verbalise* their unhelpful thinking process although not necessarily out loud. Daniel Siegel, Clinical Professor of Psychiatry at UCLA, describes this method of *labelling* our thinking processes as "name it to tame it." His book *Mindsight* (2013) integrates brain science with the practice of psychotherapy drawing on neurological research. Siegel tells us that when we use *words* to describe and label our thought processes, we activate the language centres in the left hemisphere of our brain which has a soothing effect on the right hemisphere that is more closely linked to the sometimes emotionally turbulent subcortical areas. I sometimes provide this explanation to clients when they wince at the prospect of completing tedious forms and having a better understanding of what is "going on underneath the bonnet" as one individual described it, which is often sufficient motivation to follow through with the task. Gerard also finds this explanation helpful and we part on good terms.

When we meet the following week, Gerard has dutifully completed his diary and as predicted, every worry recorded is hypothetical. I ask if he has learned anything from this exercise. He describes two insights that surprised him. Gerard imagined that he worried incessantly about every aspect of his life. The diaries revealed that certain recurrent themes have emerged and that most of his worries revolve around these. As I had discerned from his previous lengthy diary, his worries tend to focus on his wife's and his own health, job security and the as-yet undisclosed worry about his daughter. He has also managed to discover how one worry can lead to another and that if this process continues unchecked, he can spend hours engaged in hypothetical worry and suffer the consequences of constant anxiety. I probe him about this last comment as it sounds as though Gerard has managed, if even slightly, to detach from the worry process. This surprises me given Gerard's outburst the previous week emphasising his belief that he is unable to control his worrying. His response surprises me even more.

"I've tried practicing mindfulness meditation to help with my anxiety in the past but it's never helped. I just couldn't sit there for twenty minutes at a time focussing on my breathing and "noticing my thoughts". The problem was that all of my thoughts were worries and I'd become even more anxious trying to practice mindfulness because I didn't have anything to distract my mind. But the one thing that helped a little bit was what the instructor called "walking mindfulness". She encouraged us to go for a walk and focus on five things we could see, four things we could hear, three things we could feel, two things we could smell and, if possible, one thing we could taste. I hadn't practiced that approach for ages but this week whenever I noticed that I was worrying and labelled it, I used it as a prompt to focus on my senses in the same way that I was encouraged to do during mindful walking and I was surprised to find that I got some respite, even though it was fleeting. I remembered that stick figure drawing you did last week and what you'd said about how we find it difficult to be in the present moment. I tried to pull myself back into the present moment through my senses."

I am delighted that Gerard has managed to make this connection himself, and it reminded me that very often therapists forget to explore potential resources that clients already possess and that can be utilised in therapy. I encourage Gerard to persevere with his new-found approach and that continued practice will yield results.

"Every time you notice yourself worrying and manage to detach from this process by focussing on your senses, you are strengthening neural pathways that, if you persevere, will help you to take back more control over your worry. Think of it like this, it's a bit like doing reps with weights in a gym: every time you label the worry and detach from it, you strengthen the pathway."

Gerard thinks this is a reasonable approach and agrees to persevere. I also encourage him to practice *worry postponement*. If he struggles to detach from a particular worry, he can schedule a time in the day to give it his full attention and then focus on what he is currently engaged in. He agrees to try this approach but expresses some scepticism.

"I will try to do these things but I can't go for a walk every time I feel anxious."

It's a fair question and I explain that he can come up with a range of distractions that can help to pull him back into the present moment and we spend some time listing these. After a quarter of an hour, he has a range of strategies to use at work, including screen breaks and conversations with colleagues, at home focusing on listening to the radio and interacting with his daughter and finally in bed when he can't sleep due to worry when we agree that he will try listening to an audiobook. Now I have to turn our attention to the major part of Dugas and Robichaud's protocol for GAD that I have been using (2007), namely, helping Gerard to overcome his *intolerance of uncertainty*.

According to Dugas and Robichaud, intolerance of uncertainty can be regarded as the "fuel" for worry, and there is something almost existential about this assertion. Towards the end of the 19th century, the German philosopher Friedrich Nietzsche (2018) proclaimed that "God is dead" and considered atheism to be humanity's liberation from the tyranny of Christian religion. But with this freedom came the terrifying realisation expressed by existentialists like Jean-Paul Sartre that the universe is a meaningless place for the individual without any moral causality at work. Everyone has to assume responsibility for the choices they make and bad things can happen to good people for arbitrary reasons. Perhaps the rise in secularism within modern Western society has increased this existential angst and intolerance of uncertainty. The cure, according to Dugas and Robichaud, is to inure ourselves to this angst by developing *tolerance of uncertainty*. It makes sense from a clinical perspective. As we have seen in Chapter 2 when we encountered Robert's depression, one of the hard lessons of CBT is that we need to deliberately submit ourselves to physical and psychological discomfort not only to over-come depression and anxiety but also to inoculate ourselves against their onset. As we shall see in subsequent case studies, continued avoidance of uncertainty and the anxiety it provokes leads in some individuals to an ever-shrinking comfort zone that, in cases of agoraphobia, becomes so diminished that the person is afraid to step outside their front door. I explain the concept to Gerard but in far less florid terms and ask for his response. He recognises that a number of his behaviours can be described as *approach strategies* like seeking reassurance from his wife or work colleagues, checking emails at least three times before sending, and *avoidance strategies* such as avoiding taking the car to the garage, procrastinating about submitting reports until the last moment. I put this to him.

"So the main issue that you want help with is reducing your worry and anxiety. There are two possibilities: increasing your tolerance of uncertainty or increasing your certainty that nothing bad will ever happen to you. Which strategy have you been using up until now?"

"I can recognise that some of the things I do like the ones we've just discussed, are an attempt to make sure that nothing bad happens. But a lot of the time I just spend worrying about what *might* happen."

"That's absolutely right. But you've mentioned previously that one of the reasons you worry so much is that it will prevent you from making mistakes at work, that you'll be alert for any health problems you and your family might experience, that you'll prevent your daughter coming to harm. It seems that this type of worrying is an attempt to figure out any potential danger that *might* occur and is your mind's attempt to try and obtain a feeling of certainty over future events."

"Like the hunter gathers who thought about possible dangers?"

"Exactly, but do you think that continually trying to increase certainty will reduce your worry and anxiety?"

"Put like that, no, I don't think it will. But I don't know if I could ever increase my tolerance of uncertainty. I feel so ground down by it all, I don't think I could stand any more anxiety."

"It's a really tough fact of life that uncertainty is unavoidable. We don't know with any true certainty what will happen with our health, relationships, job secu-rity or anything else. Every day we're confronted with uncertainty and if we don't develop a different perspective and way of dealing with it, that uncertainty will torture us. The therapy that we're working on is based on years of research and it's effective. If you commit to it fully, I have every confidence that your worry and anxiety will reduce."

Gerard is considering what I have just said and is frowning. I begin to wonder if I could have pitched the approach in more positive tones but there isn't any way of avoiding the fact that it will take him completely out of his comfort zone. He poses an inevitable question following this explanation:

"So what do I have to do?"

"We need to work out where you're excessively avoiding uncertainty in your daily life and get you to take a few calculated risks. See what will happen if you don't engage in some of the behaviours you use to prevent bad things from happening. I know that sounds scary, but if you can stretch your comfort zone, you'll have more freedom in your life and less anxiety."

During the next quarter of an hour, Gerard and I develop a target list of experiments calculated to increase his tolerance of uncertainty. This includes:

- Send all social emails and texts without checking for spelling errors, grammar, and punctuation and without re-reading
- Exactly the same for work emails that are of minor importance
- Plan a day out at the weekend for the family rather than leaving it to his wife
- Refrain from calling his wife for reassurance when she hasn't come home at her usual time
- Reduce checking his testicles for lumps from three times each day to once a week
- Call a friend and go for a drink in an unfamiliar (but safe) bar whilst his wife babysits

You may look at this list and consider it to be quite mundane: no dramatic examples of breaking free from the tyranny of worry. But the sad fact is that GAD sufferers and worriers in general often take great pains to keep their lives as free as possible from uncertainty with the consequence of living a boring, predictable life within a stultifying, and narrow comfort zone with limited opportunities for personal growth. This impacts many areas in their lives including staying in "safe" but unsatisfying relationships, avoiding promotion opportunities and languishing in boring but undemanding jobs, and maintaining tedious but predictable routines. Unfortunately, this dire need for certainty can lead to depression or at the very least low mood to accompany the anxiety they already suffer (Shafran, Brosan and Cooper, 2013).

I notice that Gerard's list does not contain any safety routines regarding his daughter and wonder if this is a deliberate omission. He has previously mentioned worrying excessively about his daughter and I'm willing to bet that he has a number of safety behaviours to go with this fear. But his daughter remains in a zone of anxiety that Gerard is not willing to enter at this stage in therapy and I have to respect that. We put the items in order of how much apprehension carrying them out will illicit from Gerard, and I ask him to pick one to complete before our next session. I also add that the more he challenges himself with these experiments, the quicker he will make progress in therapy. He breathes a heavy sigh, and I notice that he is lacerating the skin around his cuticles with his fingernails. I hadn't noticed before but his chewed-down fingernails and the shredded skin around them bear further evidence of his constant agitation.

"I really don't know if I'm in the right frame of mind to do this. Perhaps I could come back to this when I feel more motivated, less ground down."

"Have you ever felt that level of motivation to tackle your problem?"

"Now I know what's involved, I think it's really important that I work on my motivation before I start."

"The problem is that with most challenges we face in life, waiting for motivation to tackle them is a doomed strategy. How many people do you know who want to lose weight, stop smoking or start a fitness routine who've been putting it off for years because they're "waiting for the motivation?" It doesn't work like that. If you want to make positive changes in your life that involve challenges, you sometimes have to push through when you don't feel any motivation. In fact what we're looking at now are things that you absolutely *don't* want to do let alone feel motivated about carrying them out. You could think of your anxiety as a bully that's pushing you around and dictating how you live your life. If you follow through with these experiments you'd be standing up to that bully and the more freedom you win back, the more your motivation will grow."

"So what am I supposed to do?"

"One way of approaching this is to *act as if* you could tolerate uncertainty. Do you know anyone who acts in that way?"

"My wife Christine is the complete opposite to me and she really can't understand my problem although she tries to help."

"So you could ask her how she would think and act if she were to send an email without checking—you could model her behaviour. You might have heard of this approach being referred to as "fake it until you make it.""

"I really don't think that will work for me—how could it if I've spent all my life worrying?"

"Ok, just bear with me for a moment. Can you pick up work emails on your mobile?"

"Yes."

"Good, could you turn it on please? Right, now pick an email that's in your inbox that isn't highly important and requires a few sentences for a reply. Ok, I want you to compose your reply and send it immediately—no checking, just press 'send'.""

Gerard is doing his best to comply with my request. I notice that he is frowning, his shoulders are hunched forward in a tense posture, knees pressed together, and he is absent-mindedly picking away at the scabbed cuticles of his left hand as he types the reply with his right. To my relief he presses send without any apparent checking but does not look at all happy.

"Well done. What went through your mind when you did that?"

"That my reply probably didn't make sense because I typed it in a hurry and felt stressed."

"Talking of stressed, what did it feel like physically?"

"Very uncomfortable, I can feel a slight headache coming on."

I convey my observations to Gerard about his tense posture and self-laceration whilst composing the email and he confirms my suspicion that he was totally unaware of these behaviours. As he looks down at his now bleeding fingernails, I try to reinforce the point I was making.

"So when you were composing that email with the intention of sending it without checking, you were *acting and thinking as if* you were very intolerant of uncertainty without even knowing, it was an automatic response. Your body posture and your thoughts sent a strong signal to your brain that there was some sort of threat and the result was that you experienced a spike in anxiety, hence the tension headache. What would Christine think in the same situation?"

"She wouldn't care, she'd probably think, it's just another bloody email."

"Right, and what would her body posture be like?"

"Relaxed, 'unfurled' as she calls it after she's been doing her yoga exercises."

"And this is my point. Next time you take on one of these challenges, take a moment and force yourself to think and act like Christine. Get your body into a relaxed, confident posture and tell yourself, 'It's just a bloody email'. What sort of signal will that send to your brain?"

"That there isn't a threat, everything's OK."

"Exactly, but look. If you do feel anxious, that's the point. Your trying out new things so feeling a little anxious is normal and we're building up your confidence gradually, starting with challenges that you can manage and then building up to the bigger ones. Do you remember the last time you learned a new skill?"

"Yes, paddle boarding when we were on holiday. I felt quite anxious at first but now I really love it."

"It's the same principle with what we're working on, it's called habituation. If you keep repeating the same challenge, your anxiety will decrease and go away eventually. Then you'll probably feel a sense of achievement."

Gerard studies his list reflectively, and there is a glimmer of motivation. I brief him in terms of setting up the experiments so that he can test his negative predictions about what will happen if he doesn't engage in his safety behaviours ("I'll get an annoyed response saying that my email didn't make sense") and we part company.

Over the coming weeks, something unexpected and positive emerges from our work together. Gerard engages in increasingly challenging behavioural experiments including actively problem-solving his current worries: he visited the garage and the car required some minor work that didn't cost a fortune. Little by little Gerard's confidence began to grow as he learned with each of his behavioural experiments that the dire consequences he had predicted did not materialise. But the problem still remained that his hypothetical worries persisted and his strategies for detaching from them met with mixed success. During our review of his weekly diary, I decided to explore one of Gerard's hypothetical worries in a little more depth.

"You've recorded that you're worried about being made redundant again. This crops up frequently and yet you tell me that your job is relatively secure."

"I know, when I think about it objectively I can manage to rationalise the fear but it keeps coming back."

"Could I ask you, when you worry about this possibility, what exactly goes through your mind?"

"Well, I imagine getting a call from my manager and being asked to attend a meeting with her. Then I imagine her telling me that the service is facing a reduction in funding and my job will be axed."

"And then what happens?"

"I start to think about how we would cope as a family and that I'd have to look for another job"

"So you don't go beyond the point where you've been told that you're about to be made redundant?"

"No."

"And can I also ask you, do you imagine this very vividly, with lots of images?"

"The images are quite fleeting now you come to mention it. I kind of get stuck in a loop of thinking about what I could do if I got made redundant."

Gerard's description of his hypothetical worry reveals a number of important aspects and indicates the direction that our work together will take. Following extensive research into the nature of worry a highly influential academic at Penn State University by the name of Thomas Borkovec published a study indicating that worriers engage in what he described as a "verbal-linguistic activity" with little mental imagery: they worry in words rather than pictures (Borkovec and Inz, 1990). Why is this important?—because a substantial amount of research in the field of clinical and experimental psychology suggests that imagery has a special relationship with emotion (Hackmann, Bennett-Levy and Holmes, 2011). According to these theories, worry is often a *verbal* mental process that paradoxically reduces anxiety because it prevents the worrier from confronting the disturbing images associated with their fear (Dugas and Robichaud, 2007). Gerard's hypothetical worry has very few images, and he also stops the sequence at the point when he has been made redundant and starts figuring out what action he will take. This is consistent with his positive belief about worry: that it will help him to foresee potential dangers and come up with plans to mitigate against them. The problem is that although worrying in this way reduces Gerard's anxiety when he thinks about a potential threat, he is maintaining the very behaviour that he wants to be rid of. This brings us to one of the most important components of the Dugas protocol for GAD: *imaginal exposure.*

We have identified a range of activities that Gerard has previously avoided due to his intolerance of uncertainty and he is systematically exposing herself to these. Although he finds the work challenging, it's quite straightforward because the situations are *external* and Gerard can change his behaviour towards them (sending the email without his usual checking to reduce anxiety). But what about the *internal* hypothetical worries? As these situations haven't occurred and may never occur, the only way Gerard can confront these fears is within his mind through imaginal exposure.

Dugas and his colleagues have devised this method because they discerned that worrying prevents GAD sufferers from emotionally processing their hypothetical fears and they do this in a number of ways often without being aware of it. In addition to avoiding the mental imagery associated with their fears, they often deliberately suppress worrying thoughts—Gerard has often described "blocking out" these types of cognitions. Similarly, GAD sufferers might also replace the worrying thought with a "happy" or neutral thought. For example, Gerard may force himself to switch from worrying about the possibility of being made redundant and think about taking his daughter to the park later that day. He may also engage in some form of distraction like listening to the radio, playing with his daughter, or watching TV. And he might avoid anything that triggers his worry such as media reports about redundancies. All of these responses make sense: why would anyone want to elaborate on their worst fears and increase their anxiety? But these attempts at avoidance often stem from a "fear of fear": the belief that experiencing increased anxiety is dangerous in some way and we know that Gerard suspects that ongoing stress may render him vulnerable to developing cancer.

As with other forms of exposure, Dugas and his colleagues ingeniously devised imaginal exposure as a way of helping GAD sufferers to process their worst fears but the procedure is carried out in a very specific way: they have to be exposed to the mental imagery of their worst fear *and* the physiological arousal of the accompanying anxiety. This will require Gerard, and I to develop an elaborate narrative of his redundancy fear that prevents him from jumping around in his mind and leads to his most feared conclusion. In order to do this, Dugas and his colleagues recommend using a *downward arrow* approach: constantly asking, "what might happen next." But first I have to convince Gerard to engage in this process and I suspect that he may have some reservations so I set him an objective before we meet at our next session.

"Given that the thought of being made redundant causes you such anxiety I'd like you to try something out for me. Over the following week, I'd like you to try and block out that particular worry on each alternate day but keep recording the results in your diary. What I mean is starting from tomorrow, just record whatever worry comes up spontaneously and don't do anything to control your thought processes. The following day do everything you can to block out the worry of being made redundant if it comes up. The day after that, back to spontaneous worrying and so on until we meet next week."

I don't provide a rationale, and Gerard seems amenable to trying this out. When we meet the following week, I suggest that we review his diary immediately and ask him to comment on anything significant that has cropped up during the week. He brandishes pages of detailed notes in spite of my previous admonition to keep them brief.

"What I noticed was that your suggestion to block out worrying about being made redundant was a pretty crap technique. You can see from my diary that on the days I tried to do that, it actually *increased* my worries."

"Right, that's interesting, and what do you make of that?"

"That I'll never be free of my worries."

"I want to talk to you about something called *cognitive avoidance*. It's a fancy way of describing trying not to think of something and it's a really interesting concept. What we know from research is that trying *not* to think about your worries doesn't work at all and you've just spent the last week proving that fact. But not only is cognitive avoidance an unhelpful strategy, it also makes matters worse because you get what's called an *enhancement effect*. Trying to block out any thought of being made redundant actually increased the thought you were trying to avoid. And then on top of that you get what's called *paradoxical rebound effect*. Your diary tells us that on the days you tried to suppress worrying about redundancy, the thoughts popped up all over the place. What do you make of that?"

"Am I supposed to deliberately increase my worrying about redundancy?"

"Yes and no. Let me try to explain by giving you an example. Let's say someone you know is afraid of cats. Every time they see a cat, they avoid it. What do you think they feel after they have avoided the cat?"

"I suppose they'd feel relief."

"Exactly, but what do you think the problem is with them constantly avoiding cats?"

"They'd never learn that cats are harmless and they'd live in constant fear of them. But I haven't got a problem with cats."

I'm beginning to feel that my explanation is confusing Gerard. Dugas' protocol describes fear of dogs in the example and I'm wishing that I hadn't switched to cats. I forget to talk about attempts to neutralise fears through distraction and jump to the main point I want to emphasise.

"Ok, bear with me. If you had a friend who was afraid of cats, how would you help them to overcome their fear?"

"From what I know of phobia cures, you'd expose them to the cat."

"Absolutely. So if you locked them in a room with the cat?"

"They'd get anxious but eventually their anxiety would reduce. Are you suggesting that it works the same way with my worry about anxiety?"

"Exactly. Your attempts to avoid thinking about redundancy or neutral-ise the thoughts are keeping the problem going. And you stop at the point where you've just been made redundant—do you ever go beyond that point to think of the very worst that may happen to you after you have been made redundant?"

"No and I wouldn't want to do that."

"The only way to overcome your fear is to really focus on the situation in detail and for an extended period of time."

"How long?"

"The recommendation is between 30 to 60 minutes each day for the next few weeks until your anxiety about the situation subsides."

"But I've told you before, I'm stressed enough as it is. This is just going to make me feel worse."

"Look, you were really reluctant to drop your safety behaviours and go out-side your comfort zone but you've told me that challenging yourself in this way has made you feel better about yourself. It was stressful at first but you coped. It's exactly the same with what I'm proposing and if it actually worked for you, wouldn't the initial increase in stress be a price worth paying to overcome the problems you've been suffering with for years?"

We both paused, and Gerard is silent for a moment. I'm pondering whether I have been over-emphatic and wonder if a more subtle approach would have been more effective. I have a tendency to be over-enthusiastic like this in these situations as I know that worriers like Gerard have so much mental activity going on moment by moment that sometimes it feels necessary to hammer home an important point. Eventually, Gerard sighs and asks me what he needs to do.

"What I'd like you to do is describe in detail your train of thought when you worry about being made redundant. To get us started, I'd like you to record this on your phone and then write it up between sessions. Once you've got as detailed a narrative as possible, I'm going to ask you to read it out and record it. Then every day you're going to listen to it repeatedly for at least half an hour and measure your anxiety level after each session. Any questions so far?"

Gerard looks resigned and shakes her head.

"No, let's get started. Let me just find the record function on my mobile."

"Ok, ready? Good. What's the first thing that comes into your mind when you think about being made redundant?"

"I imagine getting a call from my line manager Tess asking me to attend a meet-ing with her. I try to probe her as to the purpose of the meeting but she tells me that it would be better if she explains the situation face-to-face. I feel very anxious after I've hung up and I start to worry about whether I've done something wrong but I sense that she's going to deliver bad news that it has to do with my job. For the next two days before the meeting I find it hard to concentrate on my work and at home I feel even worse. I've told Christine about my fears and she's tried to re-assure me but it doesn't help. I lie awake in bed going over it in my mind and I can't sleep at all.

On the day of the meeting I feel sick in my stomach as I wait to be fetched from the reception area. When Tess appears and I get up, my legs feel like lead as I follow her into her office. We're sitting facing one another and she looks awkward. Eventually she tells me that she is very sorry. The service has received a substantial cut in funding for the next financial year and my job will be deleted. I begin crying and feel utterly humiliated in front of Tess. She tries to console me and tells me that she will make an appointment for me with the HR manager to discuss support that will be made available to me. I leave her office and I'm trembling, finding it hard to walk—I feel in a complete state of shock."

I notice that tears are steadily coursing down Gerard's face, and he looks quite pale but his voice remains steady as he continues.

"I get home that evening and I tell Christine the news. She tries to re-assure me and says that we'll cope, we have some money saved up that will tide us over until I can find another job. I feel a deep sense of failure, that I've let her and Clara down. I serve out the remainder of my notice period at work quietly and it seems as if colleagues are avoiding me as though I'm contaminated with bad luck or they're embarrassed and don't know what to say to me. There is no leaving party and on my last day I gather my things in a pathetic brown box and leave the building. It's a bleak, cold day and raining steadily, I feel completely alone.

Over the coming weeks I register with recruitment agencies and make multiple online applications but I keep receiving rejections or no reply at all. With each passing week I can feel my anxiety growing as we burn through what remains of our savings. Christine is trying to remain calm about the situation but I can tell that she is becoming quite concerned. We spend most of our time together in silence and she has stopped asking me how my day has been because she's probably sick of hearing about my failed attempts to find work.

After a couple of months we have to contact the bank and ask for a mortgage holiday and I feel completely ashamed of myself. The situation is putting a strain on our relationship and we argue a great deal over trivial things and it's pretty clear that Christine is losing patience with me.

During the day when Christine is at work and Clara is at the nursery, I do less and less. I have given up applying for jobs because I can't stand the rejections and I spend most of the day trying to distract myself by watching daytime trashy TV. I often go back to bed after I've dropped Clara off at the nursery and try to escape into sleep. I'm constantly exhausted because I can't sleep at night and I lie there listening to Christine breathing and think about how our lives are falling apart. I'm neglecting my appearance and although she doesn't say anything, I catch Christine looking at me with concern. I can see that she finds me pathetic because in spite of her attempts to help me, I've given in and it feels like a black cloud has settled over me.

One evening after I have put Clara to bed, Christine tells me that we need to talk. I can almost guess what's coming but when she tells me that she's met someone else and it crushes me. I cry and cry and Christine keeps telling me that she's sorry but she'll make sure everything will be ok for all of us.

Pretty soon she has moved out with Clara and our house is on the market. We have both tried to explain what is happening to Clara but she cries constantly during my visits. I've been prescribed antidepressants and now I just feel numb. I comfort eat junk food throughout the day while I'm watching TV and I've put on weight. I really don't care about my appearance now and I don't even bother to wash every day.

Eventually the house is sold and I move into a small, shabby flat. It's all I can afford because I'm on benefits now. On the day we leave the house I take stock of all the care we lavished on our surroundings, the weekends and evenings spent decorating and thinking that this would be our home for life. The flat doesn't feel like home. The neighbours play loud music and fight all the time. I try talking to them but they threaten me. The smell of their cooking permeates the flat.

Clara's nursery have asked to see me and Christine and when we meet the headteacher, she tells me that they are concerned about Clara's wellbeing as she is showing signs of emotional distress. They recommend that she sees a child psychologist."

Gerard has ground to a halt and places his face in his hands crying steadily now. I am stunned at how elaborate and specific his narrative has become now that he has allowed himself to think the worst. In my experience, clients' first attempts at this exercise are sketchy and they require encouragement to "think the unthinkable" and build in details, particularly around the emotional consequences of their fears. It seems as though Gerard has thrown open the floodgates of his imagination releasing a tormented stream of consciousness culminating in his worst fear. I hand him a tissue and wait for him to compose himself. Eventually, he remembers to switch off the record function on his mobile and gazes blankly at the floor. I realise that our time is nearly up and feel the need to carefully choose my next words.

"That was a brilliant first attempt Gerard, you did really well. I can see it was very challenging for you but if you persevere with this approach, you will see the benefits."

Gerard looks at me slightly absent-mindedly and asks,

"What was it you wanted me to do every day?"

"Find somewhere quiet and play the recording to yourself repeatedly for at least half-an-hour each day. An hour would be better if you can find the time: the more you put into this, the quicker you'll see results. At the end of each session, I'd like you to record your SUDs rating. It stands for Subjective Units of Distress scale.

Basically it's a measure of how disturbing you found listening to your narrative during the session. I'll give you a log and I'd like you to record your SUDs rating on a scale of 0 to 100 before you commence the session, at its peak and immediately after the session."

I hand Gerard the log sheet and he folds it carefully before putting it in his jacket pocket. He looks exhausted. As he gets up to leave, I add one further comment.

"Feel free to re-record your narrative and add more detail but I think what you've come up with today is more than adequate. I'm amazed that you were able to describe it in such detail for a first attempt. You certainly didn't hold back and that's exactly what's needed."

As I hold open the door for Gerard he looks up at me and says,

"It wasn't that difficult; it happened to my sister."

After Gerard has left, I review my clinical notes from our first session together concerned that I have made a crass error and overlooked the detail about his sister but I find that he hasn't disclosed anything about her. I wonder if Gerard has been afraid to even talk about his sister and his fear that he will follow the same path. Perhaps, he has a belief that talking about it or thinking about it in detail will make it come true. He is showing immense courage, and I am hoping that he will be able to persevere with the work now that it is entering the most demanding phase.

I am slightly disconcerted when I receive a text message from Gerard the following week cancelling his appointment. The details are minimal, and the text informs me that he is not feeling well but will attend at the usual time next week. I am concerned that I may have accelerated the pace of therapy too quickly and fear that Gerard may consider dropping out. After some reflection, I remind myself that this is a hypothetical worry and decide to take a leaf out of my own therapy book and let it go.

Much to my relief, Gerard attends at our appointed time the following week and even greets me with a smile, the first he has graced me with since beginning work with me. When we sit down together I ask if he is feeling better and he tells me that the past 2 weeks have been demanding. He has suffered from tension headaches, sleeplessness, and IBS symptoms but has been feeling a lot better over the past 2 days. He places his SUDs log on the table between us and I see that he has diligently recorded his level of disturbance pre, peak, and post for each imaginal exposure session. I can discern from the figures that his level of distress remained stubbornly high over the first week but then began to decline gradually and the last recording indicates almost a flatline with scores of pre: 0, peak: 10, and post: 5. I congratulate Gerard for his courage and persistence and he scans the scores before replying.

"It's been a rough couple of weeks, I must admit, but it's strange. I kept reliving this horrible nightmare scenario again and again and eventually it got to the point where the images became increasingly blurry. When I started everything seemed so horribly vivid as though I was living through it moment-by-moment. But towards the end the scenario seemed surreal, distant from me."

"What do you make of that?"

"That this approach is very painful but it seems to work."

"Could I ask you something? I don't think you mentioned your sister before."

"She's my older sister. She's ok now but she went through a very dark phase in her life."

I get the sense that Gerard does not want to elaborate on this and would not welcome any further attempt on my part to probe him for details. At this point, I'm wondering about my hypothesis that part of Gerard's initial aversion to letting his feared narrative reach its conclusion was due to some sort of magical belief that thinking about the event would make it happen. I remember attending a workshop with the Michael Dugas at Reading University in 2012 and I asked him how you determine whether clients are engaging in some form of covert neutralisation and avoidance and his answer to me was, "Sometimes you just have to have an honest and open conversation with them." He also added that it's sometimes helpful to approach the question tangentially, giving examples of experiences that other clients have described and offered them up for a response. I tentatively outline my hypothesis to Gerard.

"Some clients I've worked with have disclosed a belief that if they even talk about something they fear happening, it will tempt fate in some way to make it happen. I just wondered, does that idea resonate with you in any way?"

Gerard takes a sip of water and nods his head. Again, it doesn't seem as though he wants to elaborate. I consider my options. I know that Gerard is still holding something back concerning a fear he has about his daughter and if I can't help him to confront it, the work that we have done together may be only partially effective and render him vulnerable to a relapse.

"You've been incredibly brave in exposing yourself to that scenario, particularly if you hold that sort of belief. But I hope you can see that there are two benefits to putting yourself through this. Firstly, the exposure has helped you to process the fear and *habituate* your anxiety: you no longer find the scenario disturbing. Secondly, you'll come to see that even if you think about something bad happening in great detail, there's absolutely no way that it will make that thing come true. Once you've proved that to yourself, you'll no longer have to constantly manage your anxious thoughts all the time which must be exhausting. The one thing we haven't discussed is the worry about your daughter that you recorded in your diary. It was a frequent worry and you gave it the highest score in terms of the anxiety it causes you. Do you think we could talk about it today?"

I pause and wait for Gerard to respond—I don't want to keep bombarding him with questions at this point. He puts down his cup and looks resolved.

"I've been doing a lot of thinking about all of this over the past couple of weeks. What really made my mind up is that I'm doing this for Clara, I don't want her to inherit my fear. I know that with this condition, parents who are worriers often pass it on to their children—I want it to stop here. I have to admit something to you. Up until the past couple of weeks I checked on Clara when she was sleeping several times each night. I kept checking that she was breathing ok and it's driven Christine mad because I keep waking her up. And then one evening Clara woke up and said, "What are you doing daddy?". I could see that she was frightened and I had to calm her down—I felt so guilty. I've made a monumental effort not to check on her since then."

I decide to gently incline him back towards my question.

"And this worry you have about Clara?"

Gerard's eyes well up as he contemplates my question. Then he answers haltingly.

"Ever since Clara was born I've had this constant dread of dying. That's why I'm always afraid that I've got symptoms of cancer and why I check all the time. I want you to understand that I don't fear death itself. I've never really been religious and when I think about death I just think about oblivion, that it must be the same as before we were born—we know nothing of it then and we'll know nothing of it after. The dread I have is of leaving Clara behind with the grief I imagine she'll suffer. It's almost unbearable to think that I wouldn't be around to protect her from it. A friend of mine died of cancer a few years ago and I remember visiting her in the hospice towards the end. She was on morphine at the time and she was quite calm. One thing that she told me has always stayed with me. She said that it was a strange feeling, knowing that you would die soon because it felt as though you were mourning for loved-ones that would be left behind—almost as though it were they who were dying. And that's exactly how I feel about Clara, I fear my death all the time and I feel as though I'm mourning the loss of her ahead of time. But even more than that, I fear that I will neglect Clara in some way and that some terrible harm will come to her. That's why I feel compelled to constantly check on her at night and why I find it difficult to let her out of my sight."

I am finding Gerard's revelation a lot to take in even though I had inferred that he feared some sort of harm coming to his daughter. His fear of dying and leaving his daughter behind makes sense in the context of his morbid health anxieties. Given that Gerard has a magical belief that talking about the feared event will make it happen, he has shown immense courage in disclosing this to me. He must be experiencing an inner-turmoil between trying to suppress his morbid belief and confronting it for the sake of his daughter. If we both lose the momentum now, Gerard may never find the courage to face his worst fear. I share this concern with him and he nods, a look of sad resignation on his face.

"I think I can manage to write everything down but I won't be able to read it to myself. Can I read it to you next week?"

"Of course. You're doing absolutely the best thing for you and Clara and thanks so much for sharing this with me."

We part for a week and I am left feeling optimistic that Gerard will maintain his resolve.

When we meet the following week, Gerard's appearance has reverted to the exhausted mask he wore during the early stages of therapy. His complexion is sallow, he has dark rings under his eyes, and his fingernails and the surrounding skin are more lacerated than usual. This final task has clearly taken its toll on him and I hope that he can see it through. I don't waste time asking how he has been; that's clear enough and we both know why we are here. I wait for Gerard to compose himself and begin in his own time. Eventually, he reaches into his jacket pocket and unfolds several pages of handwritten notes. He takes out his mobile and presses the record function. My instinct is that he will only be able to recite this narrative once, and I hope very much he has mastered the recording function from his previous imaginal exposure. The scenario that he unfolds is difficult for me to bear witness to.

"I'm working from home in our attic and it's a warm spring day. Christine comes into the room and tells me that she needs to get some milk from the corner shop, we've nearly run out—could I keep an eye on Clara while she's at the shop? I tell her that's ok and I go downstairs to check on Clara. She's in the living room and playing with the antique dolls house my parents got her for Christmas, she seems really engrossed. I love the way she looks so absorbed in her play oblivious to the cares of adult life that constantly persecute me.

I'm feeling a bit lethargic and am not relishing the prospect of returning to the report I have to write when Christine returns from the shop and decide to use her absence and this welcome interruption to make a cup of coffee. I walk into the kitchen and flick on the kettle as it's already half full. I decide to put on Radio 4 while the kettle is on to reinforce the feeling of taking a short break from my tedious task. I eat a piece of chocolate in spite of my resolution to cut down on sweets. By the time the kettle boils and I pour the water over the granules of instant coffee my mood is pleasantly elevated. I pick up the mug and wander back into the living room savouring the feeling of respite from my work and consider extending it by playing with Clara even after Christine has returned and I no longer have a reasonable excuse. I reflect that every moment spent with Clara at this young age is precious and that I will never have this time with her again.

As I walk into the living room the first thing I notice is the dolls' house and Clara's absence. It occurs to me that she may have gone upstairs to her room because she wants to retrieve additional dollies to add to the ones that she has arranged on the windowsill. I climb the stairs and when I get to her room and can't find her I feel a pang of unease. I start calling her name and check the bathroom in case she has gone to the toilet but she's not there.

I can feel my sense of panic rising and leave my coffee on a cupboard in the landing dashing down the stairs calling out her name but much louder now. When I reach the hallway I notice that the front door is open and my immediate thought is that Christine must have left it open by mistake. It's at this moment that I hear the sound of a car braking violently on the street outside, tyres screeching followed by a loud bang and glass splintering as though it has come into contact with a soft object.

I rush outside of the house and see Clara's little body lying in the road motionless in front of the car—there's a thin thread of blood seeping from her mouth. The driver is standing by her, his face is white and he is trembling. He keeps saying over and over that she stepped out in front of the car—he couldn't stop in time."

Gerard pauses for a moment to wipe away the tears coursing down his face. In spite of the intense emotions that he is experiencing, Gerard is managing to live out his most disturbing narrative with a relatively steady voice. He continues.

"At this moment Christine approaches just as neighbours are coming out of their houses to see what has happened and she starts screaming, dropping the carton of milk. My immediate instinct is to try and console her but she continues screaming and begins hitting me and pushing me away.

I stand over Clara's body uselessly staring down at her until the ambulance and police car arrive. The crowd surrounding us has grown and Christine is trying to pick Clara up but the ambulance crew and police officers restrain her. Eventually they carry Clara's frail little body into the ambulance on a stretcher.

We follow the ambulance to the hospital and enter the A&E department. Everything seems in commotion and Clara is rushed through to the operating theatre. We wait together in silence and at this point I feel completely numb. Christine is sitting next to me and it seems as though a chasm has opened up between us. She sits in rigid silence looking straight ahead. I want to turn to her because I feel such turmoil but her face is cold and implacable.

We wait for hours in the neon glare of the hospital lighting with medical staff going about their business around us impervious to our suffering as we sit in silence together. My head is beginning to droop and my eye lids feel leaden with exhaustion. I catch myself falling asleep at the very moment that a young doctor dressed in scrubs approaches us with a grave expression on his face. He tells us that every attempt was made to save Clara but she died on the operating table. Christine breaks down and sobs wretchedly, convulsively. I put my arm around her shoulder in an attempt to comfort her but she pulls away from me violently.

Weeks later we attend Clara's funeral and we're sitting in the front row of the chapel. Christine is sitting next to me as the occasion requires but she is distant and cold—she will never forgive me for what has happened.

Christine has chosen Mozart's requiem and the music rises sonorously as the undertakers enter carrying Clara's little coffin. There is a floral arrangement of a white rabbit in tribute to her beloved pet. I can hear family members sobbing as the undertakers carefully place the coffin on the catafalque. The vicar begins the service and eventually it is time for me to say some words. I felt compelled to do this when we made the arrangements for the service in spite of the terrible feelings of guilt that make the burden of my grief even heavier. I feel that I have to make this gesture to Clara, to atone for my negligence. But when the moment comes and I stand before the rows of family members with Clara's coffin behind me, I try to read the words I had prepared but fall apart and the vicar has to take over. I return to the pew next to Christine and she doesn't look at me as I sit down. I watch the service draw to its conclusion through a mist of tears. The final piece of music chosen by Christine, Eric Clapton's Tears in Heaven, begins playing and is a sign for everyone to rise and leave the chapel. The curtains are closing on the coffin and I know with a sense of finality that Clara is lost to me forever."

Gerard's narrative has come to an end and he carefully folds the sheets of paper and tucks them back into his jacket pocket. He switches off the record function on his mobile and sits back in the chair—he looks exhausted. We are nearing the end of our session and I don't feel it would be appropriate for me to belabour the tasks Gerard has between sessions. After the courage he has shown today I am fully confident that he will commit to the imaginal exposure work required of him over the following week. I also don't feel inclined to comment on the content of his narrative as I want to respect Gerard's implicit need for quiet and calm following an emotionally draining session. I had expected his narrative to involve his fear of harm coming to his daughter and he didn't hold back in terms of calling up the full horror of his imagination. I ask him what he intends to do after our session and he tells me that he wants to take a long walk. I suggest that he avoids the high street and navigates towards the quiet tree-lined suburban streets 5 minutes away from our location with their grand Victorian houses and cheerful gardens. He accepts my suggestion, and I hope that he finds the early spring sunshine recuperative after his ordeal.

Due to an unforeseen work commitment, Gerard is unable to attend our next session and a fortnight has elapsed by the time we next meet. In some respects, this extended gap has been helpful as it has given Gerard more time to expose himself to his most feared scenario. As he takes his seat, I notice that he is looking fresher-faced and the dark rings under his eyes have receded. He tells me that he and his family have been taking advantage of the unseasonably warm spring weather and going on country walks together. Our room is flooded with sunshine, and there does seem to be an atmosphere of spring renewal permeating the atmosphere because Gerard is smiling as he describes his success in sticking with the daily exposures and, although the narrative still seems tinged with melancholy, it no longer disturbs him. He finds it remarkable that having imagined his worst nightmare time and again, he rarely catches himself worrying fleetingly about Clara's death.

"When I gave myself free rein to imagine the very worst that could happen and kept thinking about the aftermath, I somehow realised that I am contaminating my experience of Clara's early childhood. I need to spend every precious moment in the present with her rather than letting my fear drag me into nightmares of my own making."

Gerard has also managed to resist his night-time compulsions and no longer visits his daughter's room whilst she is asleep to check if she is still breathing. The one thing that Gerard hasn't quite got to grips with is his fear of contracting cancer and he still engages in excessive checking of his testicles for lumps although he has at least reduced the number of times he checks each day. We agree that he will end therapy with me for the time being to consolidate what he has learned during this treatment episode and get in touch if problems with his health anxiety continue. I watch Gerard walk off into the spring sunshine, and it seems to me as though at least some of the burden of his anxiety has lifted from his shoulders.

References

American Psychiatric Association. (2013). *Diagnostic and statistical manual of mental disorders*, 5th ed. Washington: American Psychiatric Publishing.

Borkovec, T. and Inz, J. (1990). The nature of worry in generalised anxiety disorder: A predominance of thought activity. *Behaviour Research and Therapy*, 28, pp. 153–158.

Csikszentmihalyi, M. (2002). *Flow: The psychology of optimal experience*. London: Harper Perennial.

Dugas, J. and Robichaud, M. (2007). *Cognitive-behavioural treatment for generalized anxiety disorder*. New York: Routledge.

Hackmann, A., Bennett-Levy, J. and Holmes, E.A. (2011). *Imagery in cognitive therapy*. Oxford: Oxford University Press.

Harari, Y.N. (2014). *Sapiens: A brief history of humankind*. London: Harvill Secker.

Nietzsche, F. (2018). *The joyous science*. Great Britain: Penguin Classics.

Shafran, R., Brosan, L. and Cooper, P. (2013). *The complete CBT guide for anxiety*. London: Constable & Robinson Ltd.

Siegel, D. (2013). *Mindsight*. London: Oneworld Publications.

Notes

* The *Diagnostic and Statistical Manual of Mental Disorders* (*DSM-5*) the bible for psychiatrists, psychologists, and other mental health workers (2013). It is used to assess and diagnose mental disorders as first step to devising an effective clinical treatment plan.
1 According to the National Science Foundation.

Chapter 4

"Why Is My Brain Doing This to Me?"

Attempting to Break Free From OCD

Sean's Story

Sean is sitting in front of me during our first session together, and he looks extremely tired. There are dark rings under his eyes, and he looks haggard and older than his 35 years. Sean has told me that he is an IT consultant for a multinational company in the city and that the job is stressful. He also explains that sleep has long been a problem because he spends hours lying in bed in the room next to his girlfriend Mary's bedroom wondering if he will kill her one day. I ask him to elaborate.

"It started just over a year ago two years after Mary and I began planning to take a year off to travel. We were both very happy with the decision because I'd become disillusioned with my job and we thought that if I could stick it out for two years, we'd have enough money to travel for a year and that would give us time to take stock of what we wanted to do with our lives. I'd been finding the work increasingly stressful and found it difficult to return after the weekend let alone after a holiday. Mary is also willing to take a break from her career and our plan is to travel around Europe in a campervan. It's a dream we'd had for a long time but then the problem started."

"We'd had some friends around for dinner one evening and Mary was clearing up next to me in the kitchen while I was loading the dishwasher. I picked up a really sharp Sabatier chef's knife that I'd used to carve the meat and. . ." Sean falters at this point and I encourage him to take things slowly.

"Mary was standing next to me and I suddenly had this image of plunging the knife into her back and I remember thinking "Oh God, what if I stab her?" "I dropped the knife straight away and ran out of the kitchen. Mary followed me and asked me what was wrong. I thought about lying but I just couldn't do it. I burst into tears and told her what had gone through my mind. We were both really shaken and I slept in the spare bedroom. I begged Mary to lock her bedroom door until the morning. And that's been our life for the past year. Mary has been incredibly understanding but it's reached a point where she is seriously thinking

DOI: 10.4324/9781003091745-5

of leaving me and that's why I decided to reach out and try therapy—it's probably my last chance."

Sean looks completely dejected, and I feel his sadness. I can tell that he is finding our session challenging and am intent on engaging him as quickly as possible. First of all, I want to explore further Sean's response to the intrusive images and thoughts about his girlfriend that he has been experiencing.

"You seem to find these thoughts and images very disturbing Sean."

"I'm absolutely horrified by them. I've always loved Mary ever since I first met her and the very thought that I could harm her fills me with dread. I've thought many times about killing myself but I know what that would do to her. Both our parents are still alive and they're getting rather frail. We haven't told them about this, it would devastate them."

I quickly ascertain that Sean has no history of harm to himself or others and I'm confident that he is not making any plans to end his life. Sean's level of distress in reaction to his intrusive thoughts and images also reassures me. With this type of OCD presentation, it's very important to discern whether the client's reactions to their intrusive thoughts are *ego-dystonic*: that they find the intrusions aversive and have no desire whatsoever to act on their thoughts. I would be very concerned if Sean were not distressed by his thoughts about killing his girlfriend as this might indicate an *ego-syntonic* response: that he might accept these thoughts as reasonable and be in danger of following them through.

I realise how distressing this conversation is for Sean and decide to go to the whiteboard and make some notes. My aim is to provide us both with a visual focus and a more analytical approach in the hope that this will enable Sean to decentre from his emotionally aroused state if even slightly. I'm also hoping that it will enable us to make sense of his experiences and provide some clues as to which direction to take in our work together. I ask his permission to do this.

"Sean, I wonder if you'd mind me jotting down a few notes on the whiteboard, is that ok? It might help us to get a sense of the problems you've been experiencing and what we can do about them. I know it's challenging for you but could we go back to the situations you described just now? You mentioned standing next to Mary holding the Sabatier knife and you had an image of stabbing her in the back?"

Sean nods and I note both of these aspects on the whiteboard. He seems a little calmer now so I press on.

"It seems to me that you're very afraid of these thoughts, that there's a danger in having these thoughts as it might make you act on them. Have I got that right?"

"Yes, why else would I have these thoughts? Perhaps I've harboured a subconscious desire to kill Mary for years and it's only now coming to the surface. I'm also worried that I'll be a danger to others, that I'm losing my mind in some way." I make a mental note that Sean's fears about acting on his thoughts are not only confined to Mary but also generalise to others. I decide to stick with exploring Sean's fear of harming his girlfriend for the moment as this issue causes him the most disturbance but I am already formulating a plan to help Sean begin to disconfirm his belief for our next session together.

"And yet you've told me that you love Mary and would never wish to harm her?"

"Yes, but perhaps it's my subconscious—I don't know." I decide not to get into a debate with Sean about his misguided assumptions concerning the working of his subconscious mind at this point.

"How much do you believe that having intrusive thoughts about harming Mary will make you act on them, on a scale of 0 to 100, where 100 means that you totally believe in this and 0 means you don't believe you're a danger at all?"

"I think, yes, 80%." I note this on the whiteboard.

"So when you experience these thoughts and images, how do you feel?"

"Horrible. I'm terrified by these thoughts and also, I feel incredibly guilty and ashamed that I could think of harming her in that way. The images are so vicious, vile."

"That sounds really disturbing—I can see how upsetting it is for you. When this happened, you mentioned sleeping in the next room and asking Mary to lock her bedroom door. Is there anything else you do to reduce the danger and your anxiety that you may harm Mary?"

"I'm very careful to avoid knives when I'm around Mary. We even eat separately and I'm seldom in the kitchen when she's there."

"Anything else? What about the thoughts? You've mentioned your fear that the thoughts will make you act, harm Mary. Do you do anything to reduce this danger?"

"I'm always aware of the possibility of these thoughts occurring and if I get even a hint, I do my very best to block them out. I'll turn on the radio and focus on that. I'll even sing songs in my head or force myself to think about our last trip abroad."

"It seems to me, Sean, that you're making a phenomenal effort to control your thoughts about harming Mary—have I got that right?"

"That's it. If I could control the thoughts or make them go away entirely, I wouldn't be a danger to Mary."

"And has that worked for you up until now?"

"No the absolute opposite. The harder I try to get rid of these dreadful thoughts, the more frequent they become along with all of the horrible images I get."

At this point, I want to begin the process of socialising Sean into one of the fundamental concepts of OCD in relation to intrusive thoughts described in clinical literature as *though-action fusion*: the belief that having a thought will

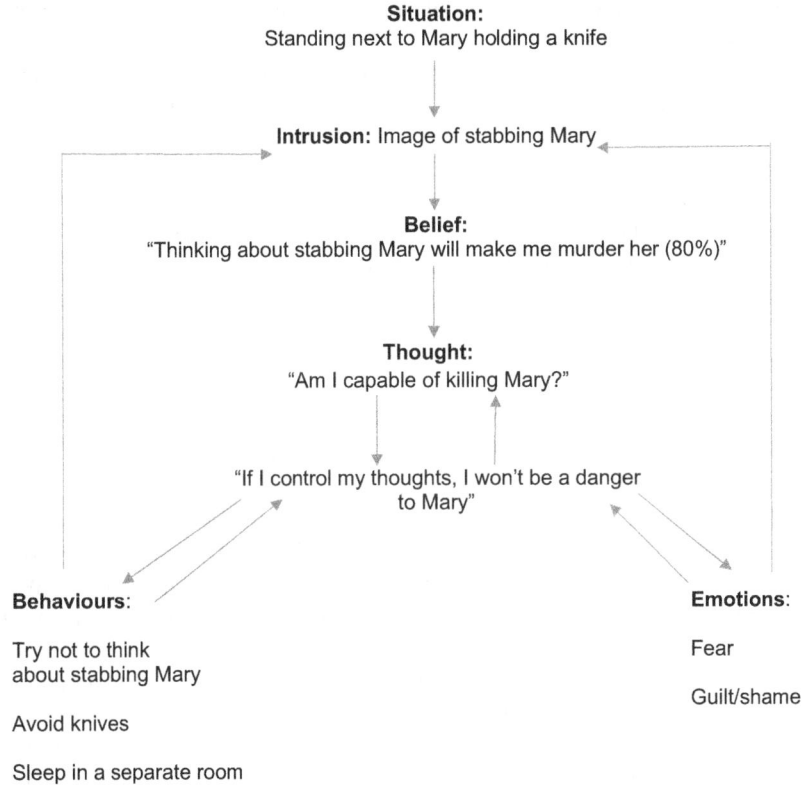

Situation:
Standing next to Mary holding a knife

Intrusion: Image of stabbing Mary

Belief:
"Thinking about stabbing Mary will make me murder her (80%)"

Thought:
"Am I capable of killing Mary?"

"If I control my thoughts, I won't be a danger
to Mary"

Behaviours:

Try not to think
about stabbing Mary

Avoid knives

Sleep in a separate room

Emotions:

Fear

Guilt/shame

Figure 4.1 Formulation of Sean's Intrusive Thoughts

lead the individual to act on the content of the thought, in Sean's case, killing his girlfriend. This phenomenon and every other aspect of OCD have been studied extensively by leading experts such as Professors Paul Salkovskis (Salkovskis and Warwick, 1985) and Adrian Wells (2008a). Their work and that of their colleagues in the field of OCD have enabled therapists specialising in CBT to relieve suffering experienced by people like Sean. I point at the whiteboard and direct Sean's gaze to the vicious cycle I have sketched against his belief that thinking about stabbing his girlfriend will cause him to kill her and his attempts to suppress these thoughts. I ask him what he makes of this and he responds tersely.

"I think you're implying that I'm keeping the problem going in some way although I'm not sure how."

Sean has become defensive, and I want to avoid any suggestion that he is delusional and responsible for his own suffering so I decide to change tack and provide an illustration. I put this to him.

"I wonder if you'd mind trying something out with me for a few moments—a little experiment? It is related." Sean concedes grudgingly, and I realise that using the whiteboard to reduce his arousal level has only been partially effective.

"Ok. I just want you to sit back in the chair, get yourself comfortable and close your eyes. Do you mind doing that for me?" Sean nods, which is a relief. I'm concerned that he may be so hypervigilant about intrusive thoughts and that he might be unwilling to close his eyes and place himself at risk. I am going to describe an unusual image to Sean and then ask him to make every effort not to think about it.

This procedure in *thought suppression* had originally been devised by the psychologists Wegner et al. (1987). They asked participants in their experiment to avoid thinking of a white bear but to ring a bell if they did. They found that participants who engaged in thought suppression were more likely to think of a white bear, and this reaction was described by them as *the rebound effect*. Therapists have developed variations on this approach presumably because they find white bears mundane. Professor Adrian Wells, for example, uses a blue giraffe (Wells, 2008b). My own personal preference is for a pink rabbit.

"What I'd like you to do Sean, for the next 3 minutes, is to try as hard as you can *not* to think of a pink rabbit. It's extremely important that if you get a hint of that image, you're to push it out of your mind." Sean opens his eyes at this point, and the expression on his face is disconcerting: a mixture of incredulity and annoyance. Nevertheless, I press on.

"Just go with it Sean. As I said, I want you to make every effort not to think of a pink rabbit. However, if you *do* think of a pink rabbit, I want you to raise your hand. OK, time starts—now!"

Sean's facial expression shifts from irritation to concentration as he engages in the task. After a few moments, he raises his hand—it's pink rabbit time. Soon after, his hand goes up again and again and several more times before the 3 minutes elapse. After he has opened his eyes and re-oriented himself, I point at the whiteboard and ask,

"Do you see the connection?"

"Yes, I see the point you are making—the more I try not to think about harming Mary, the more likely I am to experience that thought. But the thoughts are still loathsome and frightening."

"Yes, so your strategy of trying to banish the thoughts isn't working for you. The problem, if I'm understanding you correctly, is that you believe the thoughts will compel you to harm Mary. What if I could help you to learn that the thoughts you're experiencing are just that: random mental events that your mind has latched onto with no power to make you act against your will?" Sean considers this for a while and concedes that he is willing to suspend his scepticism and meet me the following week.

I begin our next session by checking how Sean has been, and we examine the thought monitoring log that he has agreed to keep for me. We review this together, and I can see that his intrusive thoughts of harming Mary have become more frequent and disturbing and also that his attempts to suppress the thoughts and images have become more desperate. He is dejected about this turn of events and shares with me the fact that he very nearly cancelled our session with the intention of abandoning therapy. I need to reassure Sean that the increase in intrusive thoughts that he is experiencing during the early stages of therapy is quite a common occurrence.

"First of all, I'm really pleased that you decided not to cancel. It must have taken you a lot of courage to come here and I really believe that I will be able to help you overcome this. Just consider what's happened this week for a moment Sean. Up until now you've been doing your utmost to keep these thoughts and images at bay with some limited success because they keep returning. But last week you were talking about them openly. It's understandable that the intrusions have increased because you've given them even more attention than usual. But as I said last week, the big problem you have is that you believe the thoughts will cause you to act on them. Let's think of it in terms of a theory that you maintain."

Just before our session together, I have re-drawn the formulation from the previous week on the whiteboard. I refer back to it and write underneath:

Theory A

"My thoughts are dangerous and will make me harm others, Mary in particular. I need to control my intrusive thoughts."

I ask Sean if I've described his belief accurately and he nods. I get him to rate the strength of his conviction in this belief, and he provides a score of 90% so I know that I have my work cut out. I then ask Sean to consider an alternative perspective.

"What would an alternative theory look like as far as you're concerned?" He looks slightly disgruntled at my question.

"I suppose you want me to say that my thoughts are neutral or something like that."

"I don't want to put words in your mouth but from what you've said, you care very much for Mary and you're very worried about harming her and perhaps others?"

"We can definitely agree on that."

"What about the insight you gained last week—do you remember?"

"You mean the more I suppress the thoughts, the more likely I am to keep them going?"

"Exactly. So if we put that together, do you think we have an alternative theory about the problem you're experiencing?"

Theory A:	Theory B:
"My thoughts are dangerous and will make me harm others, Mary in particular. I need to control my intrusive thoughts." (90%)	"I care very much about Mary and worry about harming her and other people. Trying too hard to control my intrusive thoughts is keeping them going." (15%)

Figure 4.2 Theory A & Theory B

Sean considers the whiteboard and concedes that he is willing to consider Theory B but that his level of conviction is only 15%. He looks sceptical and I need to keep encouraging him.

"That's absolutely fine—it's a baseline. Now what we need to do as part of our work together is look for evidence to disprove Theory A and strengthen Theory B."

"And how do you suggest that we go about that?"

I take a seat opposite Sean. There is a small table between us with just a box of tissues. I reach down into a plastic shopping bag I have placed next to my chair at the start of the session and drawn out a sharp 6-inch kitchen knife and place it on the table between us. It's from Tesco's basic range rather than Sabatier, but I can see from Sean's expression that he's not going to quibble about brand superiority. He is ashen-faced and rigid in the chair. I'm also feeling apprehensive. Not because I fear that Sean will harm me, I'm absolutely certain that he won't. My concern is that he may find the next intervention too anxiety provoking and abandon therapy altogether. If I had told Sean in advance that I would be bringing a knife to the session, chances are that he wouldn't have turned up. However, I do owe him an explanation and a rationale for introducing a very important component in treating OCD—Exposure and response prevention.

"I'm sorry to spring this on you Sean but this is really important. We've established that you believe your thoughts are dangerous and will compel you to act on them. I'm absolutely convinced that isn't the case but I need to prove it to you. What I'd like you to do is think "I will stab Steve.""

Sean's eyes don't move from the knife sitting on the table between us as he answers me.

"I'm not going to do that."

"Sean, I'm 100% confident that if you think those words, you will not harm me. I've trained thoroughly in CBT and I have treated many clients with similar problems to you. This isn't something I've dreamt-up, it's based on many years of research. If you want to free yourself from this problem it's really important that you take this next step."

Sean nods slowly and says "OK." I feel a surge of relief and ask him to rate how much anxiety he is feeling on a scale of 0 to 100 right now. He tells me 95%.

"OK Sean. What I need you to do is say out loud, 'I will stab Steve.'"

Sean says the words very tentatively, and I encourage him to keep repeating the statement. Once I am confident that he is in the flow of repeating the words, I instruct him to continue silently in his mind. As he continues to do this, I check Sean's anxiety ratings frequently. I really feel for him as he is clearly experiencing intense anxiety, and his hands are trembling slightly. But eventually what I'd hoped for begins to happen and his anxiety starts to decline. After 20 minutes of exposing himself to what he believes to be a lethal thought, Sean's reported level of anxiety has dropped to 30%, a significant level of reduction and enough for us to conclude the exposure.

I ask him the obvious question, what did he make of the experiment? He is still looking at the knife so I remove it and put it back in the shopping bag. After a few moments of reflection he answers,

"That was absolutely awful but I can see why you did it. I thought you were crazy at first but I'm really surprised at how my anxiety came down. I still feel shaky but at the start it felt as though I was going to have a panic attack."

"Well done Sean, you did brilliantly and you might feel a bit shaky for the next hour or so with all of that adrenaline in your system but it'll fade. So, we've got our first piece of counter-evidence to Theory A." I write on the whiteboard:

"Can I just check, what's your strength of conviction in Theory A now?" Sean considers this for a few moments.

"85%"

Theory A:	Theory B:
"My thoughts are dangerous and will make me harm others, Mary in particular. I need to control my intrusive thoughts." (85%)	"I care very much about Mary and worry about harming her and other people. Trying too hard to control my intrusive thoughts is keeping them going." (15%)
Evidence against:	**Evidence for:**
I thought repeatedly, "I will stab Steve" for 20 minutes with a knife in front of me and did not act on the thought.	

Figure 4.3 Theory A & Theory B with Evidence For and Against

"That's a good start but we're going to have to keep working on it if you want to overcome this problem. The best thing we can do is to set up further experiments like the one we've just carried out so that you can chip away at this belief. You've seen how, if you confront your fear and nothing bad happens, your anxiety level will reduce and you'll learn something really important: that your thoughts won't compel you to harm anyone, especially not Mary. But we need to do this in a systematic way. What I'd like to do with you now, is map out what we call an exposure hierarchy. But before I do that, I want to show you something."

At this point, I draw the following diagram on the whiteboard:

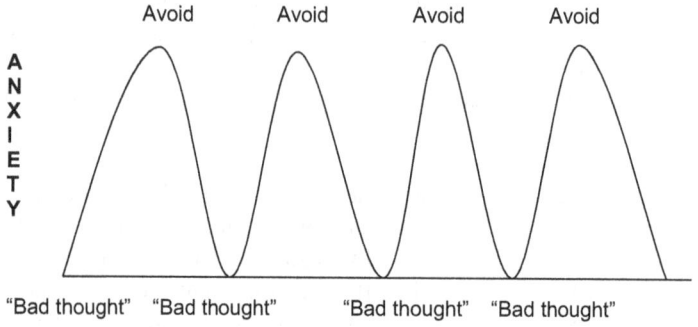

Figure 4.4 Thought Avoidance Graph

"At the moment, every time you experience an intrusive thought about harming Mary or anyone else, you push it out, you avoid it. What happens when you do that?"

"My anxiety goes away, temporarily."

"That's exactly right. The problem you have is that you experience temporary relief from your anxiety but you've never given yourself the opportunity to *disprove* the fact that if you stayed with the thought, nothing bad would happen. Now, what do you think would happen if you stayed with the thought and even forced yourself to keep repeating it like you did with me just now?"

"Well, based on what you just shown me, my anxiety would reduce but I don't think it would go away completely."

Sean is still understandably sceptical, but I am encouraged by the concessions he is making. I rub out the diagram on the whiteboard and draw another simple graph:

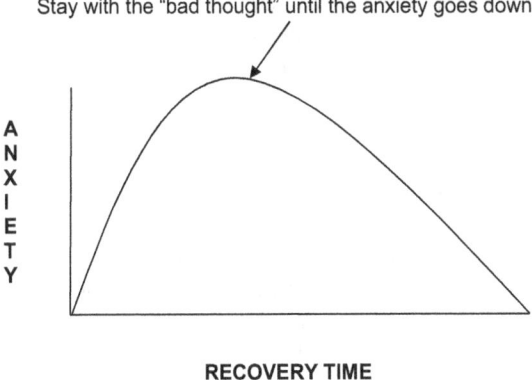

Figure 4.5 Thought Exposure Graph

"In actual fact, if I kept you here repeating the thought about stabbing me for another hour or more, your anxiety would flatline—you'd probably become bored thinking it. And you'd start to realise, bit-by-bit, as your 5% reduction indicates, that these thoughts are *harmless,* they won't lead you to hurt anyone." Sean studies the whiteboard for a few moments and then responds with further healthy scepticism.

"OK, I get the point you're making. If I kept thinking about stabbing you, my anxiety may go down. But what if we meet tomorrow and I have the same thought? I'm back where I began."

"That's a really good point and I have one more diagram for you in answer to it. What do you make of this?"

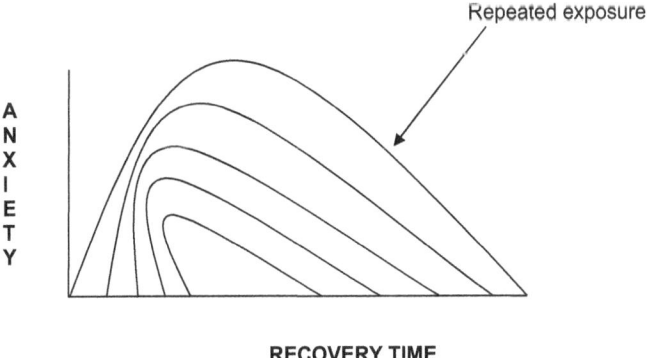

Figure 4.6 Repeated Exposure Graph

"I'd have to keep returning to that particular thought and exposing myself to it until I'd convinced myself it was harmless." Sean's expression now indicates something closer to reflection than scepticism, and I want to keep the momentum going.

"That's right Sean—you've got it. We have to carry out these exposures in a systematic way recording your level of anxiety each time so that you can see that there *is* a reduction. And we also need to keep checking that this work is leading to a similar reduction in your belief that your thoughts are dangerous and will make you harm others. But we have to target other intrusive thoughts including the ones you find most challenging. What I have in mind is something called an *exposure hierarchy*. It's like a ladder where you start off with a thought and activity that's challenging. Once you've overcome it, you move up to the next challenge. Would you be willing to work with me on this?"

Sean looks apprehensive but nods cautiously. I rub out the diagrams on the whiteboard and turn to him.

"OK Sean. We can put these down in any order but we're looking for thoughts and activities that would cause you to feel anxious on a scale of 0 to 100 where one hundred is the most anxiety you could possibly experience. Have you any idea of what 100 would represent for you?"

"Based on what we've just done, thinking a similar thought repeatedly near Mary would represent 100."

"What about holding a knife while you're thinking it and being near Mary?"

"I don't think I could do that under any circumstances. You can put that down if you want, but I don't think we'll ever get to it."

"What about me? What number would you put on holding a knife and thinking that you'll stab me."

"The thought of that makes me quite anxious right now. I'd say that's around 40."

"What about standing over me holding a knife while I have my back to you thinking that you'll stab me?"

"I would find that very challenging—that's probably a 70."

We carry on in this way until the end of the session when Sean's hierarchy looks like this:

THOUGHT/ACTIVITY	ANXIETY RATING
Holding a knife standing near Mary and thinking of stabbing her	100
Standing in the kitchen with Mary where there are knives and thinking of stabbing her	80
Sitting next to Mary in the living room and thinking of stabbing her	75
Sitting at the other end of the sitting room from Mary (where there are no knives) and thinking of stabbing her	70
Standing over Steve with his back to me thinking that I will stab him	60
Holding a knife facing Steve thinking that I will stab him	40
Sitting opposite Steve with a knife on the table between us thinking that I will stab him	30

Figure 4.7 Sean's Exposure Hierarchy

Sean has revised his anxiety rating downwards for the third item in the hierarchy. I ask him how he has found the session. He takes a photograph of the hierarchy on his mobile phone and says:

"Strangely and against my expectations I feel slightly hopeful but very anxious. There's some sense in what you've said but I'm not sure that I'll be able to follow through all of the items on the hierarchy."

I do my best to maintain the positive tone of the session and encourage Sean to come up with evidence to support Theory B between sessions and we agreed a time to meet.

When we resume working together the following week, I am pleasantly surprised by the vigour with which Sean throws himself into his exposure hierarchy. He manages to hold a knife and think of stabbing me until his anxiety level drops to 5 so I make a decision to jump to the next level and ask him to follow my instructions.

"OK Sean, you're doing brilliantly and I want you to get the most out of this session. I'm going to sit in this chair with my back to you. I want you to hold the knife pointing down just between my shoulder blades. Have you managed to do that? How's your anxiety level?"

"I'm feeling very uncomfortable."

I can hear the anxiety in Sean's voice but I take the decision to keep pushing. We have a limited number of sessions together and I have to make sure that he makes significant progress each week within the limits of his tolerance.

"You can do it Sean—that's good. Now that you've got the knife in place, I want you to keep thinking, 'I will stab Steve'. Say it out loud a few times and then in your head."

"I will stab Steve!"

"Good, excellent—keep repeating that in your head. Now what I want you to do is imagine the blade going into my back and blood gushing out down my shirt."

I'm wondering if I'm pushing him too hard at this point when I feel a very slight prick between my shoulder blades and feel my own anxiety level start to creep up. I take a breath and try to rationalise. I tell myself that Sean is trying so hard to engage in the exposure that he's actually resting the tip of the blade on the fabric of my shirt. It's not a *particularly* comforting thought but I realise that if I show any sign of fear, Sean may lose faith in the confidence I have espoused for the method which may have dire consequences for our therapeutic relationship.

It's at times like these when I feel confronted by my own hubris in therapy and I'm reminded that CBT therapists aren't always rational under pressure no matter what image they like to project. Just 2 weeks ago I was carrying out a similar exposure exercise at a railway station with a client who was terrified at his intrusive thoughts about jumping in front of a train. I had spent weeks preparing him for this moment following thorough risk assessments. But as we both stood at the edge of the platform on that grim, rainy November morning with the train thundering down the tracks towards us, the thought occurred to me, "what if he actually jumps?"

The slight pressure of the knife tip remains and is now accompanied by a minute tremor. I ask Sean to report his anxiety level, and he tells me that it is 80. I don't want to speculate as to my own anxiety rating at this point and concentrate on calm breathing. How rational do you have to be as a therapist?

I remember attending a workshop with the previously mentioned Professor Salkovskis at the Maudsley Hospital in south London. He's a very entertaining lecturer and uses various flourishes to illustrate teaching points like licking the sole of his shoe to demonstrate how to challenge fear of contamination in clients. His other party trick is to instruct a hall full of therapists to write down the name of a loved one followed by the incantation that they will be killed in an accident later that day. He gleefully tells members of the audience, including a number of senior CBT therapists, to leave behind their slips of paper on a table at the front of the lecture hall and he observes that at most events, a significant number fail to do so. My slip of paper was also absent that day. It is time to check in with Sean again.

"What's your anxiety level now Sean?"

"40"—relief, I can calm down now.

"Well done Sean, keep going."

Eventually, Sean's anxiety rating drops below 20, and as we're nearing the end of the session I call a halt to the exposure and put us both out of our misery. Once he has regained his composure, Sean parts company with me in good spirits and we agree a time for our next session.

I have little time for reflection after we part company as I have booked therapy sessions with clients back-to-back until I get a short break after 2 pm. I am sitting at my computer hurriedly eating a sandwich whilst typing up clinical notes when my mobile rings and I answer it absent-mindedly. A woman says to me in a terse voice,

"Hello, is that Mr Sheward?"

"Yes, that's me."

"I'm Mary McCray, Sean's partner."

"Hi, how can I help?"

"I don't want to get off on the wrong foot but would you mind explaining what the bloody hell you think you're doing with Sean?"

Mary sounds polite but very angry at the same time and I realise that Sean has been regaling her with descriptions of my therapeutic methods, much to her horror. I can understand her apprehension as they have both been afraid of Sean's intrusive thoughts about stabbing Mary and now, as far as she can discern, I'm actively encouraging Sean to put a knife to my back. It occurs to me too late that I should have discussed with Sean the issue of how much to disclose to Mary about his treatment at this stage. Fortunately, Sean has given me consent to discuss treatment with Mary; otherwise, I would have had a potentially awkward situation in which I would have had to decline her request for an explanation on the grounds of client confidentiality. I try to make my voice sound as sane and professional as I can.

"Hello Ms McCray. I'm really sorry that this has come as a bit a surprise to you but what I'm doing with Sean is part of a NICE approved treatment plan based on years of research." This doesn't do anything to placate her.

"It seems thoroughly irresponsible to carry out therapy using a knife when Sean has constant thoughts of killing me. Where on earth do you people get your ideas from?"

I decide that I don't stand much chance of reassuring Mary over the phone. Maybe I can convince her to attend the next session with Sean and spend some time explaining the treatment process and rational. I may be using up some of Sean's precious clinical time but if I can't get his partner on-side, her antipathy towards my methods could undo any progress he is likely to make in therapy.

"I can understand your concern Ms McCray and that the methods I'm using may seem unorthodox. What I'd like to do, if Sean's in agreement, is for you to attend the next session with him. That will give me an opportunity to give you a full explanation of what we're doing in treatment and, hopefully, put your mind at rest." There is a pause at her end and then she says,

"Alright, I'll come along. But I'm not particularly happy about this situation."

I reassure her as best as I can and hurriedly prepare for my next session. As an after-lunch treat, I am carrying out exposure work with a client who has a diagnosis of OCD with fear of contamination. I will be putting my hand down the toilet and then eating crisps with my un-washed fingers to model the exposure exercise for the client—you really have to "walk the talk" in this job. I need to quickly check the condition of the toilet. There are limits to how far you can push someone on their exposure hierarchy, my own included.

The following week I meet Sean who is accompanied by Mary. She looks rather formidable, and I remember him telling me that she is a senior marketing director. Sean's expression is one of wry amusement and I wonder if he senses my slight apprehension about the conversation I am due to have with his partner.

I invite them into the therapy room and have arranged the seats in anticipation. I ask Mary to tell me what specifically she is concerned about regarding Sean's treatment and she responds in a more measured tone than in our exchange over the phone the previous week.

"My concern is, and has been for quite some time, that Sean has an unconscious desire to kill me and this is now coming to the surface. Your treatment methods may cause him to act on this desire."

There it is again, that mention of "unconscious desires" although Sean used the term "subconscious." I decide to probe her on where she gets this notion from.

"It would really help me to know what you mean by Sean's 'unconscious desire'. How do you think that works?" Mary fixes me with a direct gaze.

"My mother is a psychodynamic psychotherapist, I know about Freud's theories of the unconscious mind."

That explains it. Sigmund Freud (2005) famously maintained that forbidden feelings and desires often remain repressed and inaccessible to the conscious mind because they are forbidden or dangerous. Freud believed that these unconscious desires occasionally reveal themselves in dreams, what he referred to as the royal road to the unconscious, or "Freudian slips." These theories become problematic when applied to OCD intrusive thoughts about being a paedophile, harming a loved one or blaspheming in church because they imply that the individual harbours these secret desires when in actual fact they are horrified by the thoughts and would rather die than act upon them. I know I need to tread carefully as I don't want to get into a theoretical argument with Mary. I ask Mary about her mother, and she reveals that she trained in the 1980s and is now retired.

"Freud was an amazing pioneer and many of his ideas are still relevant today. We've come a long way in developing our knowledge of how OCD works. We know that it's common for most people to experience random disturbing thoughts like standing by the platform's edge and suddenly wondering what it would be like to jump in front of the train." I notice Mary paying particular attention to my last remark and risk a question.

"Has that ever happened to you?"

"As a matter of fact it has."

"And do you think it was evidence of an unconscious desire to kill yourself?"

"Now you put it like that, no not at all. I was concerned that I'd had the thought and moved back from the platform."

"Could I share something with you?"

I pass Mary a side of A4 titled Normal Intrusive Thoughts (Purdon and Clark, 1992). It's a table therapists often share with clients suffering from OCD and who are disturbed by what they consider to be abnormal cognitions. The table shows the results of research findings from a survey of 293 students (198 female, 95 male), none of whom had a diagnosed mental health problem. The column on the left shows the type of intrusive thought, and the two columns on the right show the percentage of men or women who said they had experienced that particular thought. Thoughts are wide ranging and include having sex with an unacceptable person (48% female, 63% male), jumping in front of a train or car (25% female, 29% male), and breaking wind in public (31% female, 49% male).

"Can I ask what you make of these findings?" I notice that Sean is studying the figures closely along with Mary. She responds.

"What jumps out at me is that there's such a high percentage of these people who had thoughts about harming a family member (42% female, 50% male), and some of them actually thought of stabbing a family member (6% female, 11% male)."

"That's right. Now what do you think the difference is between how they responded to these thoughts and how Sean has reacted?"

"I'm not entirely sure."

"The difference is that they may have been temporarily bothered by these thoughts but they were able to dismiss them for what they were: random unpleasant thoughts. Sean, on the other hand, is horrified by these thoughts because he loves you very much and fears harming you. This isn't evidence of an unconscious desire to kill you, it's the exact opposite."

"Perhaps, but why are you getting him to hold a knife to your back and think about killing you?"

"I have to prove to Sean conclusively that his thoughts will not compel him to act against his will. What do you think Sean?" Sean has been silent since we came into the room together. After pausing reflectively he replies.

"I'm beginning to think you're right. I'm slightly less anxious about having these thoughts. In fact I brought the thought up deliberately when I was in the living room with Mary and for the first time the thoughts started to lessen of their own accord. I felt anxious at first but when I stopped battling with the thoughts, I began to feel calm much to my surprise." Mary is studying Sean closely and says,

"I didn't realise that's what you were doing." There is no anger in her voice and she has taken his hand whilst looking into his eyes. Her next question is directed at Sean and takes me by surprise.

"Would it help you to overcome this dreadful problem if you held a knife over *my* back and thought about killing me? I'd do it for you if it would help."

I can see tears appearing in Sean's eyes as he nods. It seems that the three of us are in tacit agreement about what to do next as I place the knife on the table. Mary positions herself with her back to Sean and he stands behind her with the blade poised between her shoulder blades. I ask him for his anxiety rating and he reports 90%—his face is flushed. My instinct is that I don't have to ask Sean to say the words aloud and I trust his motivation sufficiently not to be concerned that he is neutralising the thought of stabbing Mary covertly. We continue for the next half an hour in this way with Sean reporting on his anxiety levels frequently until they decline to 20%. We have 10 minutes left for the remainder of the session, and I invite them both to stop. They sit back in their chairs looking exhausted, but touchingly they are holding hands. At the end of the session, I accompany them to the door and we agree that Sean will attend unaccompanied the following week.

When I meet Sean at our next session, his demeanour seems lighter; he is smiling. He informs me that he and Mary have shared a bed for the first time since his problem began. He also tells me that they have prepared meals together using their sharp Sabatier knives.

"And the thoughts?"

"They still come and go, a lot fainter now and I'm barely bothered by them at all. That last session was a breakthrough for me. Being able to do that with Mary while you were with us gave us both courage. We now realise that my reaction to the thoughts was a perverse indication of how much I love Mary and her decision to render herself so vulnerable was a gesture of her love towards me."

In our final session, we develop a relapse prevention plan detailing subtle signs that may indicate that Sean is slipping back into previous patterns of thinking and acting with contingency plans for dealing with these possibilities. I feel confident, however, that they will both be ok.

Two months later I receive a postcard from Salzburg in Austria. It depicts a beautiful view of the alps in the distance. It is from Sean and Mary and they inform me that they are travelling Europe in their camper van—the sabbatical that they had hoped for.

References

Freud, S. (2005). *The unconscious*. London: Penguin Books.

Purdon, C. and Clark, D.A. (1992). Obsessive intrusive thoughts in nonclinical subjects. Part 1 content and relation with depressive, anxious and obsessional symptoms. *Behaviour Research and Therapy*, 31, pp. 713–720.

Salkovskis, P.M. and Warwick, H.M.C. (1985). Cognitive therapy of obsessive-compulsive-disorder—treating treatment failures. *Behavioural Psychotherapy*, 13, pp. 243–245.

Wegner, D.M., Schneider, D.J., Carter, S.R. and White, T.L. (1987). Paradoxical effects of thoughts suppression. *Journal of Personality and Social Psychology*, 53, pp. 5–13.

Wells, A. (2008a). *Cognitive therapy of anxiety disorders—a practice manual and conceptual guide*. Chichester: Wiley.

Wells, A. (2008b). *Metacognitive therapy for anxiety and depression*. New York: The Guilford Press.

Chapter 5

"I'm Not Being Rude—I'm Terrified of You"

Breaking Through the Isolation of Social Phobia

I receive an email enquiry with contact details indicating that this particular client wants help with social anxiety. When I make the initial phone call, I soften my voice accordingly. To my surprise, this approach elicits an unexpectedly brusque and assertive response.

"Can I ask you, what are your qualifications? Are you a psychiatrist? I specifically wanted to be seen by a psychiatrist."

I am somewhat taken aback by this as he doesn't seem at all socially anxious— quite the opposite. I explain that I am a senior CBT therapist and have been practicing for several years. He pauses and thinks about this before replying.

"Ok. I'll see how it goes. But I might ask to be seen by someone more experienced depending on how things work out during our first session."

The appointment is now confirmed, and I begin to worry about the session with my new client next week. In spite of years of practicing CBT, I still have to guard against a tendency to worry and doubt my professional capability. Having supervised many therapists over the years, I see this tendency in others too: many of us are people pleasers with occasional imposter syndrome that gets triggered by the way our clients interact with us.

The day comes around quickly, and I meet Martin for the first time and invite him to take a seat. It's normal practice for the clinician to sit nearest the door for safety reasons. There are, however, situations in which it's more appropriate to offer your client the seat nearest the door, if they suffer from claustrophobia, for example, or are highly anxious because of their trauma presentation. Martin does not look at all anxious but insists on sitting near the door. My immediate sense is that he is imposing control over the situation and literally putting me in my place.

As I cover some administrative details I am discretely observing Martin. In terms of his appearance, he is tall, well-groomed, and very smartly dressed in a designer suit. The cut of his suit suggests many hours spent in the gym, and his body language suggests outward confidence although interestingly I notice that he is not making direct eye contact with me and there is something defensive about the way he shifts position in the chair folding his arms and crossing his legs. He reaches into his pocket and hands me the clinical questionnaires that he has completed prior to our session.

DOI: 10.4324/9781003091745-6

An important part of CBT therapy involves measuring client's symptoms and tracking their progress each session. One of the methods I use to measure recovery is by getting clients to complete a range of clinically validated questionnaires throughout treatment. I ask everyone is asked to complete a Minimum Data Set (MDS) each session irrespective of their particular presentation. The MDS includes a measure of depressive symptoms (PHQ9), anxiety symptoms (GAD7), and a measure of work and social adjustment, namely, the impact the client's problems are having on their work, home, leisure activities, family, and relationships. In addition to the MDS, I ask clients to complete a specific questionnaire measuring symptoms of their primary presentation. In this instance, Martin has completed the social phobia inventory (SPIN) and I can see that he has scored 68—the absolute maximum. Martin's scores on the MDS indicate moderate symptoms of depression and anxiety. I draw his attention to the SPIN score, and he nods slowly unfolding his arms and uncrossing his legs. He takes a deep breath and begins to describe the problems he has been experiencing, all of the time avoiding eye contact with me and directing his narrative to the table between us.

Martin is a senior manager within an international IT company; it has taken him a great deal of hard work and self-sacrifice to get to this position. He describes his climb from what he calls "humble beginnings." He was born in Sheffield, and his father left home when Martin was 3. His mother had to bring him up without support from his dad and had to do a cleaning job in the morning and evening to bring money into the home. He was a bright child and managed to get into grammar school but was really ashamed of the marks of poverty that were apparent to all the other middle-class pupils in his class. Getting away to university with a full grant enabled him to reinvent himself, to a certain extent. It was a more socially diverse environment than his grammar school and he developed strategies for managing the shyness he had experienced throughout his childhood and adolescence. He achieved a first-class degree and won a graduate entry position with his current employer and was sponsored to take part in their fast-track MBA programme.

As Martin is talking I am surprised by his candour, given his initial behaviour towards me, but now his narrative is pouring out of him almost unchecked as though he has been carrying it around like a burden and wants to be relieved of it. Still he addresses the table between us.

"I was doing really well in my career until last year. There was a decision to second a senior manager to my department from our sister company in Germany. The idea was that he would observe how I manage my end of the operation in the UK to see if he could integrate any knowledge back into his own division. Right from the start I didn't get a good feeling about this bloke. He sits in meetings watching me and hardly says anything. There's something inscrutable about him and he's not very approachable. It started gradually but I became increasingly self-conscious in meetings when it came to my turn to make a contribution and I began to lose confidence in what I had to say. The other thing is that public speaking is a major part of my role but a few months ago I had to give this presentation. I was really nervous but managed to make a start but I couldn't carry on. It felt like I was having a panic attack and I had to make an excuse and leave the room. Now I dread having to give a presentation and I've been able to avoid it by delegating to more junior staff but I don't know how long I can get away with it. I'm sure my team notice my anxiety and they probably think I'm weak, that I've lost the plot. It's got to the point where I have to take beta blockers before a meeting to manage my nerves. The thing is, because I no longer trust what I have to say in meetings, I spend hours in the evening beforehand preparing for questions that might come up. I'm probably working 16 hours each day and I'm exhausted—my sleep's suffering too. And. . . . "

Martin tails off, his face flushed. He draws a breath before continuing.

"And it's not just work. I split up with my girlfriend last year—I don't think this situation helped our relationship. I've got a group of friends I've known since Uni and they invite me to parties but I'm even beginning to dread them because I feel uncomfortable talking in a group."

"How do you manage Martin?"

"To be honest, the way I manage the situation is to drink a load and maybe do a couple of lines beforehand." It's clear that Martin has fallen into the trap of using cocaine, alcohol, and beta blockers to manage his anxiety in social situations and give himself artificial confidence, although even these measures don't seem to work for him. My usual sense of urgency around clinical time passing is prompting me to intervene and "get to work" but my instinct is to use this session for Martin to tell his story, to unburden himself of the huge weight that he has been carrying around for months. Unless he feels heard, Martin will not be able to listen to me. But I am not passive in the process—I am constantly formulating Martin's problem asking the occasional question and providing the odd prompt.

As we draw near to the end of the session, I gently indicate to Martin that our time is nearly up and ask him how he has found our first session recalling his caveats for continuing therapy with me. He looks drained but makes eye contact with me for the first time.

"Well, you're super-easy to talk to. Yes, happy to come back next week."

And that will be my immediate challenge for our next session as I haven't socialised Martin into the CBT approach we need to adopt together and I have risked giving him the impression that therapy will consist mainly of offering him a safe space to ventilate his feelings. That approach would provide him with relief in the short term but do nothing to help him overcome his problems. I resolve to brush up on Professor David Clark and Dr. Adrian Wells' (1995) CBT protocol for social phobia before our next session as it is the gold standard for treating Martin's presentation.

According to Professor Clark (2001), other phobias persist because of avoidance, which is why exposure is an important part of therapy. If you keep running away from the mouse you are afraid of, you will never discover that it's terrified of you and poses no danger whatsoever. But people with social phobia, he observes, have to enter feared social situations because of the nature of modern society. And social situations can include parties or workplace meetings: in fact any interaction with other human beings. We can relate the model to Martin's situation. Part of Martin's problem arises because of the way he *processes social situations*, imposing excessively high-performance standards on himself ("I have to sound intelligent and authoritative"). He has conditional beliefs about the consequences of his performance ("If I show any signs of anxiety, my team will think I'm weak").

It seems he has negative beliefs about himself and I am wondering to what extent his childhood experiences play a role. I need to move on to the next part of the model which is described as *processing the self as a social object*. This means that when Martin believes he is being scrutinised by others and evaluated negatively, he will monitor his performance and interpret his negative thoughts and feelings as evidence of what his team think of him.

I am beginning to feel a great deal of sympathy for Martin. Most people I know, myself included, have suffered from social anxiety on occasion even though they wouldn't meet criteria for a diagnosis of social phobia included within the *Diagnostic and Statistical Manual of Mental Disorders* (*DSM-5*) *the* bible for psychiatrists, psychologists, and other mental health workers (2013). This frequently happens in the workplace which can be a competitive environment where performance is evaluated and fitting in with the team is an essential requirement. But this type of anxiety is also common in social situations such as parties where there is a different type of performance anxiety that triggers fear of being rejected by the group.

Most emotions that we experience are assumed to have an adaptive function, and evolutionary psychologists (Leary, 2001) speculate that being hypersensitive to any sign of disapproval from the group prevented our ancient ancestors from being banished into the wilderness and we have inherited this fear of becoming a social outcast in the same way that the "fight or flight" response has been passed down to us through the generations over thousands of years. More recent findings from a study using neuroimaging (Cascio et al., 2015) suggest that the same parts of the brain are activated when we feel physical pain or *social* pain—the sub-genual anterior cingulate cortex and the dorsal anterior cingulate cortex. The suggestion is that these brain areas produce the same physical sensations of pain whether we have cut our finger or feel excruciating embarrassment at the prospect of social rejection. This makes sense from a survival point of view as we remain social animals and highly interdependent on one another.

When we meet the following week, Martin seems more amenable and apparently no longer feels the need to assert himself as the alpha male in our relationship. On reflection, his initial aggressive behaviour may have been an over-compensation for his anxiety about meeting me and disclosing what he perceived to be his "weaknesses." I immediately address the issue of socialising Martin into what he can expect from therapy going forward, that it won't just be an opportunity to get things off his chest. and that we will be working on his problem together in a structured way and he will have a number of tasks to complete between each session. To my relief, he seems happy with this business-like approach and I outline our first task: formulating Martin's problem on the whiteboard to obtain a better understanding of how his social anxiety gets triggered and what he does in these situations. This approach is particularly helpful when working with clients who suffer from social anxiety as the focus of attention shifts from themselves to the whiteboard as they may find the therapist's gaze uncomfortable, particularly during the first few sessions. I notice that Martin is still avoiding eye contact although not as much as the previous week. I ask Martin for a recent typical example.

"That's easy. We had our monthly team meeting yesterday and I nearly lost it again."

"What do you mean by 'lost it'?"

"I became so anxious when it was my turn to speak in the meeting, I thought I was going to have a panic attack. I nearly made an excuse and left the meeting."

As Martin is speaking, I make notes on the whiteboard.

"What was it about the situation that was so nerve-wracking?"

"It's like I said last week, *he* was there watching me in that inscrutable way he has and I just knew that I had to sound authoritative in front of my team or risk losing their respect. It's a very competitive environment and I can't afford for them to think of me as a weak leader."

"What was going through your mind as you were speaking and you felt yourself getting anxious?"

"I thought to myself, I *know* they can see I'm anxious—it must be so obvious."

"What symptoms did you notice?"

"I could feel myself getting red in the face and I started to sweat. My heart was pounding away and my hands felt shaky."

"What did you think other people in the meeting could see?"

"My fear."

"Sure. What I mean is how do you think you looked in front of the others?"

"Red-faced, sweaty and shaky. Someone not holding it together."

"And did you do anything to disguise your anxiety?"

"I remember gripping hold of my pen to disguise the shaking and I clamped my arms to my sides in case they saw the sweat patches. I'd taken my jacket off because I knew I'd get hot."

I finish writing and we contemplate the formulation on the whiteboard. I ask Martin what he makes of it.

"It makes sense, I can see how it links together but I'm not sure what you mean by safety behaviours."

"From what you've told me, you do a few things to draw other people's attention away from what you think they can see: you notice that you're sweating so you clamp your arms to your sides; you feel your hand shaking so you clutch your pen. We call these "safety behaviours" because they're aimed at reducing your anxiety. Unfortunately, they can actually make things worse. Can you see how?"

"Not really, no."

"OK. Well if you're feeling hot due to the anxiety, clamping your arms to your sides will make you even hotter and increase the likelihood that you will sweat. Clutching your pen tightly will magnify any tremor and both of these behaviours will probably increase your self-consciousness in the situation."

"Ok, what do I do about it?"

Martin's blunt question forces me to think hard about how I can structure treatment to help him with his problem. One of the most important aspects of David Clark's protocol for treating social phobia is setting up a situation in which the client is videoed interacting with a stranger (usually another clinician acting as a "stooge"). This is because they have a "felt sense" of what they look like to others based on their symptoms of anxiety. Martin's blushing, perspiration, and slight tremor probably go completely unnoticed by his team and the taciturn German colleague but due to his subjective experience of these symptoms, Martin creates an image in his mind of himself as a trembling, sweating blushing nervous wreck. The only way to disconfirm his belief that he looks this way to others is to present Martin with visual evidence of how he actually appears—hence the video recording. The challenge I have is that the situation needs to be sufficiently anxiety provoking; otherwise, Martin will discount it.

I'm willing to bet that getting him to chat for 5 minutes with any "stooge" I can arrange won't work as Martin's fears about speaking in public are linked closely to his concerns about losing authority within his team. Martin has talked about his social anxiety generalising to other situations such as parties, but based on what I have seen, he is able to manage day-to-day interactions with strangers even if his eye contact wavers with me occasionally. I explain my dilemma and ask if there is any possibility of someone videoing Martin either giving a presentation or speaking at a meeting. Martin's immediate reaction is to reject the idea on the grounds that recording his performance in public would make him even more self-conscious. However, after a few moments of reflection, he concedes that it might be worth pursuing and he is desperate to overcome his problem. Martin has an idea. He will be attending a less formal "keep in touch" meeting with a smaller group during the week. Presenting at the meeting causes him considerable anxiety but not to the same extent as his monthly team meeting. Martin's plan is to get his PA to discretely film him on her mobile phone when he presents at the meeting. He will tell her that a friend wants to set up a similar forum in his company and the recording will provide him with a flavour of the meeting. Delighted at Martin's creative solution, I instruct him not to watch the recording until we are together at our next session. I also ask him to engage in his usual safety behaviours for the first half of the meeting and then drop them completely for the second half.

When we meet the following week, Martin has loaded the recording on his MacBook so that we will be able to view his performance on a larger screen. My own preparations have included obtaining a red paint swatch because I want Martin to predict which shade of crimson his blush will register on the screen. He opts for "Pomegranate Punch," whereas I feel confident that his colour won't go beyond "First Blush." I get him to model for me how much he will tremble during his presentation and ask him to estimate how noticeable his perspiration will be (his conviction rating is 75%). He tells me that he felt very anxious during the meeting, and an added worry was the fear that someone would notice his PA recording him and conclude that he had really lost the plot. Before we watch the recording, I add a few more detailed instructions.

"What I'd like you to do Martin, is run a 'mental video' of your performance and see in your mind's eye how you appeared to others during the presentation." Martin closes his eyes for several moments and does this.

"Next, when we review the recording together, I want you to imagine that you're watching someone else—you need to be completely objective in your evaluation of what's taking place."

Martin nods and presses "play." As we watch the recording, a huge grin spreads across his face and he begins to laugh. If his perception is similar to mine, we are both watching a confident, professional-looking executive providing a briefing. There is a minor difference between the first and second parts of the presentation: when Martin drops his safety behaviours he seems more relaxed and spontaneous. I ask him what he makes of his performance and he shakes his head again smiling.

"It's really unbelievable. All that fear I'm feeling at the time—I can't see any of it."

"And if you can't see it, what about your audience?"

"No, you're right. I really get it."

Martin's reaction illustrates why it is so important to carry out this type of experiment during the early stages of therapy. He now has a more positive image of how he appears to colleagues and can take this into subsequent meetings when he is called upon to present. He also realises that his safety behaviours have been counterproductive and that he needs to drop these altogether.

When we meet the following week, Martin reports a significant improvement in his performance at meetings. Although he still feels anxious, his confidence is growing as he knows that his colleagues can't see the physical symptoms that he experiences. We also discuss what Martin refers to as his "paranoia" around what his team and the German colleague think of him, and I introduce him to the concept of *mind reading*. This is a very common mistake that people make in social situations, particularly when they become anxious and feel compelled to check if others have noticed their anxiety. Closely studying facial expressions and body language when anxious is extremely unhelpful as the information available is ambiguous and will often lead to misinterpretation. When Martin looks hard enough for evidence that others have noticed his anxiety, he makes faulty inferences that inevitably confirm his fears.

Over the next two sessions, I am encouraged by the progress that Martin is making in the workplace and he is now "pushing the pendulum": deliberately making mistakes and long pauses during presentations and learning that none of these actions draw a negative response from his audience as he had previously predicted. He is, however, less successful when engaged in social interactions outside of the workplace and is despondent at how the shyness that blighted his adolescence has returned its grip on him. We review different situations, and it becomes clear that Martin believes that others will find him boring, particularly women, and he engages in a number of safety behaviours. These include mentally preparing what he is going to say, monitoring his delivery to determine whether what he has to say sounds "interesting" and carrying out a mini post-mortem to evaluate how he came across to his audience. When he isn't tying himself up in mental knots like this, he holds back at the edge of conversations and his main contributions are asking other people questions rather than asserting his own opinions. When he becomes particularly anxious during conversations with others, he will make an excuse to go to the toilet, get a drink, or leave the gathering early. He always drinks alcohol before and during the event, but fortunately he is abstaining from taking cocaine as he realises that this makes him feel jittery and induces him to talk "verbal diarrhoea." I am interested to know why Martin's new-found confidence around public speaking in the workplace isn't helping him at parties or other social gatherings.

"I've been thinking about that. When I'm at work, now that I'm getting better at managing my nerves, it's different. I generally know what I'm talking about and it's like I've got a script to refer to. I can generally predict the kind of things that will come up at meetings but parties are different."

"It sounds from what you've told me that you put a lot of pressure on yourself."

"Yeah, that really is it. Do you want to know something crazy?" Martin is blushing slightly and then he adds:

"It's got so bad that I can't even have a piss in front of anyone. When I try, I freeze up and have to pretend and then sneak back into one of the cubicles later on."

Martin is describing a condition called *paruresis* also known as *shy bladder syndrome*. It often afflicts men when they try to urinate in public toilets because they become tense at the very moment they need to relax. Women also suffer from this condition although their fears are about being heard rather than the subject of scrutiny. What Martin is describing seems consistent with his social anxiety, and he tells me that this has come back to haunt him from adolescence along with his shyness. I want to pursue the issue of Martin's teenage years as he keeps referring back to them in relation to his social anxiety. I ask him what he thinks the connection is and he suddenly looks very sad.

"It's strange, this memory keeps coming back to me—I thought I'd put it behind me. When was at Grammar school, I was friends with a boy called

Peter Price. He was very popular with all the other pupils including the girls. His parents were quite well off. His dad was a dentist and his mum was quite snobbish. It was the complete opposite to my own circumstances. My mum was a single parent and had two cleaning jobs so money was always short. While Peter always wore the latest fashion, I only had one jacket. One day Peter invited me to his 15th birthday party and I really wanted to go because I had a crush on a girl called Susan from our class and I knew she was going. I got the feeling that he had reservations about inviting me but might have been too embarrassed not to.

When I arrived at his house, Peter's mother answered the door and I could see from her face that I wasn't welcome. I went into the living room and there were small groups of friends from school and his other friends that I didn't know. I saw Susan and really wanted to talk to her but kept putting it off. I tried to join a group but I just hung back at the edges pretending to take part but feeling more and more self-conscious. After a while when no one involved me in the conversation, I felt stupid and wandered off on the pretext of going to the toilet. As I walked past the dining room, I heard Peter's mother speaking to him in a quiet voice. She was asking him why he had invited me and that he'd created an awkward situation with me being there. Her next comment was like a slap in the face. She said, "What do you think Susan's parents would think if they knew you'd invited him?" All this time Peter had remained silent and I quietly walked back into the living room. Someone had put music on and suddenly Susan saw me entering the room. She and another girl I didn't recognise were looking at me and whispering to one another and then Susan said, "Would you like a dance Martin?" I didn't feel like I could decline and she started moving around me gracefully while I tried to dance awkwardly and mimic her movements. Everyone was watching and then she said, "Martin, you look as though your marching not dancing!" and everyone fell about laughing just as Peter walked in the room, joined in and took Susan's arm. I could see all of their faces laughing at me and I felt totally humiliated. I just run out of the room and out of the house."

Tears are streaming down Martin's face, and I can see that the man in the room with me is no longer the smart, confident IT executive but an adolescent boy who has been completely crushed. This gives me an idea.

"Martin, I want you to try something. Close your eyes and go back to Peter's living room as though you're there right now as your older self. Tell me what you can see, where's young Martin?"

"I'm in the living room and Susan has just put the music on. There's a slightly spiteful smile on her face as she's looking across at young Martin. He looks really awkward and uncomfortable, slightly scruffy compared to the other kids."

"How do you feel towards him?"

"I really feel for him—he looks so vulnerable: he doesn't deserve this."

"What's happening now?"

"Susan's dancing around him and it's agonising to watch, he's so clumsy. Now she makes her remark and everyone's laughing at him including Peter who's taken Susan's arm."

"What do you want to do?"

"I want to help him."

"Ok, do it!"

"I've put my arm around his shoulders and I'm shouting at them. I tell them that they're a bunch of arseholes and should be ashamed of themselves. They look shocked and they're backing away from us."

"Now I want you to be young Martin. Older Martin's got his arm around you. What do you need from him?"

"I want him to take me away from here. We're walking out of the living room and we meet Peter's mum whose come to find out what the shouting is about. Older Martin turns to her and calls her a lousy snob and says that she's beneath contempt. She's lost for words and we leave the house. Martin slams the door on the way out."

"What else do you need from him?"

"He's telling me that things will work out for me. I'll get to university and get a brilliant job, that my life's going to be an amazing journey and that what I've had to put up with is going to make me a better person."

Martin is silent now, tears glistening on his cheeks. He remains sitting this way for several minutes, and I decide not to prompt him. He will come back into the room when he is ready.

The reason I have undertaken this approach is that there is good evidence (Lee and Kwon, 2013) that *imagery rescripting* can have a significant effect in helping clients overcome social anxiety. As I mentioned previously, Clark and Wells (1995) maintain that people who suffer from social anxiety experience negative images of themselves when they are the focus of attention. A study by Hackmann, Clark and McManus (2000) also found that these images are often linked to disturbing early memories (e.g. being humiliated by a teacher in front of the class) but most people, just like Martin, are unable to make this link. When Martin has regained his composure, I ask him how it felt to help his younger self and also experience support from his adult self.

"It was really strange. It felt as though I was actually back there and the feeling of humiliation was excruciating. But it felt as though I'd righted a wrong when I stood up to them. I know it sounds like a bit of a cliché, but it feels as though something's shifted within me, like I've settled an old score that needed sorting."

"It's interesting that the memory has come back during this recent period of vulnerability that you've been experiencing at work. What do you make of that?"

"It's exactly like you say, when I'm feeling vulnerable the memory comes back, particularly in social situations. It feels as though I'm that shy, awkward teenager again. When I'm feeling confident about my life, the memory doesn't come up."

"So now you know where the feeling comes from, what do you need to do?"

"I need to override it and act more confidently, remind myself that I'm not young Martin anymore and that I've come a long way."

I'm interested to see if Martin will be able to sustain this sense of defiance towards his anxieties when he is next in a social setting and ask him if there are any forthcoming opportunities. A friend has invited him to a party Saturday evening, and he was considering making an excuse as he won't know many of the others. After some negotiation, Martin agrees that he will attend and make a concerted effort to drop his safety behaviours including monitoring his performance, staying silent, or asking questions. He also agrees to undertake a major challenge: completely abstaining from alcohol before and during the party. We set this up as a behavioural experiment to test Martin's negative predictions about how other people at the party will respond if he drops his safety behaviours and speaks up at least five times during the evening to complete strangers. Martin is 70% certain that if he speaks up within the group, the others will ignore what he has to say and carry on the conversation without acknowledging his contribution. He is also 40% certain that someone will make an excuse and leave the conversation.

Before we end the session, I remind Martin to draw on one of the skills I had taught him to use to overcome his fear of public speaking: maintaining an external rather than internal focus of attention. If he is to overcome his shyness at social gatherings, it will be essential for him to draw his *internal* focus away from the negative voice in his head and the feelings of anxiety in his body to the *external* focus of what he can see and hear around him. Martin has been diligently practicing this shift of attention during conversations with colleagues at work and has found that, when he manages to move away from self-focus, he can actually get carried away in the flow of the conversation. He agrees to practice this and jokes that although he will be abstaining from alcohol at the party, he will nevertheless try to "get out of his head."

As we part company I congratulate him on how he took care of young Martin during the session and encourage him to keep pushing himself outside of his comfort zone. He smiles wanly and replies,

"It feels like work rather than leisure. I've had all of that stress during the week and now I have to inflict even more on myself over the weekend."

"It may feel that way at the moment but if you stick at this, the goal is for you to eventually enjoy yourself socially."

When we next meet, Martin reports that the party he attended had been a mixed experience. He managed to drop his safety behaviours and engage in a number of conversations after overcoming his initial apprehension and was surprised to discover that rather than snub him, the people he had not met before showed a genuine interest in what he had to say and he managed to get into the flow of the discussion. The memory of "young Martin" at the party did not come up. He found it rather boring drinking orange juice all night but was rewarded with a clear head on Sunday morning and went for a run. I congratulated Martin for making such good progress and expressed surprise at his slight despondency. He acknowledged that he could now "hold his own" at social events but the sticking point came back to his ongoing problem.

"I still feel very self-conscious when I'm talking to women, particularly when I find them attractive. I got talking to someone and in spite of everything you've taught me, I started to feel uncomfortable during the conversation and made an excuse to break off."

"Do you remember what you were thinking?"

"That she probably thought I was boring."

"And was there any *objective* evidence for this?"

"Nothing obvious. At first the conversation seemed to be going ok but then I started thinking, what if I run out of things to say?"

"You don't seem to be the kind of person who's often at a loss for words. Was there anything else?"

"I suppose it was because I thought that she might end the conversation and walk off—I really didn't want that to happen."

"Why?"

"Because it would prove that I had been boring her and I would have felt humiliated."

"So you got your defence in first and made your excuse to end the conversation?"

"You could put it like that."

"I wonder what she made of you walking away like that. Perhaps she thought you'd found *her* boring."

"She seemed very confident."

"So do you, outwardly. The point is, it's often very hard to know what people are thinking and feeling in social situations because they're so ambiguous. But this fear of rejection seems to be a big problem for you."

"It really is. I've never had the confidence to ask someone out on a date. Of the few relationships I've been in, the other person has made the first move or we've been introduced. I do feel quite stuck as I don't want to stay on my own."

"What's the worst thing about being turned down if you ask someone for a date?"

"I don't think I could stand it—I'd fall apart. When I even contemplate doing it, I feel terrified."

"That's a really strong reaction. You mentioned the other week that you've done skydiving. Are you telling me that you find the prospect of asking someone for a date more terrifying than throwing yourself out of a plane?"

"Yes, I'd rather jump out of a plane than ask someone for a date any day of the week."

"Is that you talking or 'young Martin'?"

"I know the point you're making and it probably does go back to that party with Susan, but I'd hate to feel that humiliation again, I think it would crush me."

I pause for a moment and calculate how much time we have left during the session. I realise that my lunch break follows this session so that I can risk running over slightly. I turn to Martin.

"How much do you want to overcome this problem?"

"I'd do anything."

"OK, grab your jacket. We're going for a walk down the high street."

Martin looks at me inquisitively but does as he is told. It's a mild spring day so I don't have to fetch my jacket. As we wander down the high street, I explain my plan to Martin.

"It seems to me that you have this belief that you won't be able to tolerate the pain of rejection if you ask someone for a date and they decline. That's where you're stuck. How would it be if you learned that you *could* tolerate the feeling and that it's nowhere near as bad as you're making it out to be in your head?" Martin looks uncertain as we turn off the high street onto a less busy road with a parade of shops. We have passed a dry cleaner's and I have spotted an attractive young woman behind the counter. I draw Martin to a halt outside the paper shop next door.

"Ok Martin, what I want you to do is go into that dry cleaner's and ask the young woman behind the counter for a date." The colour drains from Martin's face at this point.

"There's no way I could do that."

"You said that you'd do anything to overcome your problem—this is the only way. Do you trust me?" Martin nods hesitantly. I wonder if he felt like this when he was about to jump out of the plane for the first time—he'd probably prefer it right now.

"Alright, let's set this up as an experiment the same way we've done for all of your other assignments. This is all about testing your hypothesis and learning from it. What's the worst thing that you think will happen?"

"She'll be angry with me, tell me to piss off or something."

"On a scale of zero to one hundred, how much do you believe that's likely to happen?"

"100%!"

I then attempt to operationalise Martin's prediction that he will "fall apart" and "won't be able to stand" the rejection. This proves to be a little trickier but we settle on an estimation that the intensity of his embarrassment will be 100% and will take at least 2 hours to subside. Now it's the moment of truth.

"But I don't know what to say."

"We'll make that part of the experiment, that you'll figure out something to say spontaneously."

I give Martin a pat on the back and a slight shove in the direction of the dry cleaner's and he enters hesitantly. I cross the road and take out my mobile pretending to take a call whilst observing from a discrete distance. I am intrigued to see that Martin and the young woman in the dry cleaners are engaged in what appears to be a friendly conversation with much smiling from both parties. Eventually, he raises his hand in a parting gesture and she responds in a similar manner as he leaves the shop. Martin sees me and crosses the road with a beaming smile. I ask him what happened as we walk back towards the high street.

"Well, I started asking about how long it would take to get my suit dry cleaned."

"Very good opening gambit—what happen then?"

"It felt like I'd broken the ice and my nerves levelled off a little. Then I just asked her if she'd like to go out for dinner with me."

"And how did she respond?"

"She was really nice about it. She said that she already had a boyfriend but that it 'lovely' that I'd asked."

"So your prediction that she would be angry with you proved to be false. How intense is your feeling of embarrassment right now?"

"I don't think I feel embarrassed, just a bit jittery because I'd worked myself up so much before I went into the shop. I'm amazed that I actually feel quite good because even though she turned me down, she was really nice about it."

"So what have your learnt?"

"That it was nowhere near as bad as I'd made it out to be in my head."

Martin looks slightly flushed with elation and I want to capitalise on this positive outcome by getting him to really "push the pendulum" before our next session.

"So your homework this week is to ask as many women as possible for a date and practice getting rejected. This is a form of exposure and if you engage with it, you will overcome both your *fear* of rejection and learn to tolerate any feelings of embarrassment or awkwardness after you've been turned down."

I am drawing on what the famous therapist and founder of rational emotive behaviour therapy Albert Ellis (2004) described as *shame attacking*: deliberately doing something that would under normal circumstance make you feel embarrassed in order to lower your inhibitions and develop confidence. He famously admitted to shyness as a young man when it came to asking women for dates. His remedy was to ask one hundred women for a date in one day and although they all declined, he rapidly overcame his shyness. This is my aspiration for Martin. He agrees to accept the challenge as we discuss how he can maximise opportunities for rejection. It transpires that Martin has been to a bar in the area with friends that hosts Ceroc lessons and dancing once a week. He recalls watching people take part with envy whilst he kept himself to his group of friends. It occurred to him at the time that learning to dance would be a great way of meeting people if only he could overcome his inhibitions. He also noticed that all of the people taking part in the class appeared to be single. Martin sets himself the considerable challenge of attending the beginners' dance class *and* asking someone for a date if the opportunity arises.

The following week Martin is in a buoyant mood when we meet and I ask him how the assignment went.

"It went really well. I went to the dance class and at first I was really nervous because I didn't know anyone there. I must admit, I had a couple of drinks beforehand to get me in the mood and I noticed that most of the others were in the same situation in that they didn't know anyone. The instructors were really good. They made everyone feel relaxed and kept getting people to change partners when we practiced the basic dance moves so it really didn't matter if you were there on your own. And because we were all focused on the dancing, it was easy to relax and chat in between. After the lesson they threw the floor open and I managed a very shaky dance with one of the girls I'd been partnered with. It seemed like a natural progression to buy her a drink afterwards and then I just asked her."

"Asked her what?"

"I asked her if she'd like dinner with me and she said yes. I've been on my first date with her."

"So you didn't do what I'd asked you to do."

"What do you mean?"

"You didn't practice getting rejected." Martin laughs and shakes his head. I ask him what he has learned from this.

"It's amazing but the very fact that I went there with the *aim* of getting rejected completely took the pressure off of me. Admittedly, I'd had a couple of drinks but I wouldn't have been able to ask someone for a date before then even if I'd downed a bottle of wine."

I congratulate Martin and I ask him if there are any remaining issues that we need to address in our work together. He hesitates in his reply and looks quite bashful. I wonder what has prompted this response given the unexpectedly rapid progress he has made and probe him gently.

"I can see from your expression that there's something on your mind. I want to make absolutely sure that I've helped you as much I as can before we reach the end of therapy. If there's something that we haven't covered, it would be better to address it now rather than end therapy and wish you'd addressed it."

Recently, Martin's eye contact with me had improved markedly to the extent that he is consistently able to hold my gaze. He is now looking at the table between us as he had done during our initial sessions. I wait for him to make his decision and he begins slowly, his face slightly flushed.

"The thing is, although it was a first date, things got quite physical. Anyway, Kate, that's her name, made it clear that she wants to sleep with me on our next date."

"Do you feel ready or are things going to quickly for you? If you need to take things at a slower pace, you need to tell Kate."

"Part of me is delighted, she really seems to like me and I'm keen on her. It's just that, I'm anxious."

"That's perfectly understandable. You haven't been in a relationship for quite some time. That's why it might help to take the pressure off you if you ask Kate to take things slowly."

"Even if we took it slowly, I don't know if it would help."

"Why?"

"This is a really embarrassing thing to admit to . . . but I always worry about . . . size."

The expression on Martin's face tells me that this disclosure has taken a great deal of effort and courage. I feel the intensity of his embarrassment. Dr. Abraham Morgentaler is a urologist and Harvard Professor and an expert in treating issues of male sexuality. In his book (2015) *The Truth About Men and Sex,* Morgentaler maintains that most men believe that their penises are smaller than average. Professor David Veale, who we will meet in Chapter 8 when confronting vomit phobia, conducted an amazing study in 2014 (Veale et al., 2014) aimed at addressing this common anxiety in men. In the imaginatively titled paper *Am I normal?* Professor Veale and his colleagues published findings from the biggest review of measured penis size amongst 15,521 subjects and determined that:

- The average length of a flaccid penis was 9.16 cm (3.6 inches)
- The average flaccid circumference was 9.31 cm (3.66 inches)
- The average length of an erect penis was 13.24 cm (5.21 inches)
- The average erect circumference was 11.66 cm (4.59 inches)

Veale and colleagues noted that many men express concern about penis size when they attend urologists or sexual medicine clinics even though their size falls within a normal range. The concern is often described by clinicians as "small penis anxiety" or "small penis syndrome" and can even be diagnosed with body dysmorphic disorder when this preoccupation becomes excessive. Interestingly, a *New York Times* article (Stephens-Davidowitz, 2015) published around the same time as Veale and his colleagues' survey indicated that men Google more questions about their penis than any other body part and one of the more common questions was about size. There are also varying hypotheses around whether or not easy access to pornography has increased small penis anxiety due to the fact that male actors are untypically well-endowed and present "distorted data" for viewers. Veale and his colleagues (Veale et al., 2015) address this issue in another clinical paper, *Sexual Functioning and Behavior of Men with Body Dysmorphic Disorder Concerning Penis Size Compared with Men Anxious about Penis Size and with Controls: A Cohort Study,* noting the fact that as pornography websites are amongst the most frequently visited in the world, watching pornography may not be linked to small penis anxiety as it has become the "norm" although the jury is still out as to its negative influence or not.

So, at this point I delicately outline Professor Veale and his colleagues' valuable findings to Martin and he raises his eyebrows in appreciation. It seems that the statistics have put his mind at rest as he is now showing an interest in the technical aspects of the research. However, I return to the issue of Martin taking the development of his new relationship at a slower pace if possible to enable him and his partner to get to know one another a little more before they go to bed together for the first time. Before we part company, we agree dates for our final two sessions.

Later in the week, I receive a phone call from Martin and he informs me with regret that due to work commitments he will need to conclude therapy ahead of our last two sessions. He thanks me for the work we have carried out together in therapy, and I praise him for the courage he has shown and diligent application throughout. Before he concludes the call I can't resist the temptation to ask how his date went, less out of prurient curiosity and more as a means of establishing whether he has maintained his clinical gains. Martin laughs and tells me that everything worked out fine.

"I took Viagra—I didn't want to leave anything to chance."

A mixed success then. Martin made significant progress in therapy because he was able to drop all of the safety behaviours that had previously maintained his social anxiety. I just hope he hasn't acquired a new long-term safety behaviour.

References

American Psychiatric Association. (2013). *Diagnostic and statistical manual of mental disorders*, 5th ed. Washington: American Psychiatric Publishing.

Cascio, C. N., et al. (2015). Narcissists' social pain seen only in the brain. *Social Cognitive and Affective Neuroscience*, 10(3), pp. 335–341.

Clark, D.M. (2001). A cognitive perspective on social phobia. In: W. Ray Crozier and Lynn E. Alden, eds., *The international handbook of social anxiety: Concepts, research and interventions relating to the self and shyness*. West Sussex, England: John Wiley & Sons Ltd.

Clark, D.M. and Wells, A. (1995). A cognitive model of social phobia. In: R. Heimberg, M. Liebowitz, D.A. Hope and F.R. Schneier, eds., *Social phobia: Diagnosis, assessment and treatment*. New York: Guilford Press.

Ellis, A. (2004). The road to tolerance. In: *The philosophy of rational emotive behaviour therapy*. New York. Prometheus Books.

Hackmann, A., Clark, D.M. and McManus, F. (2000). Recurrent images and early memories in social phobia. *Behaviour Research and Therapy*, 38, pp. 601–610.

Leary, M.R. (2001). Social anxiety as an early warning system: A refinement and extension of the self-presentation theory of social anxiety. In: S.G. Hoffmann and P.M. DiBartolo, eds., *From social anxiety to social phobia: Multiple perspectives*. Needham Heights, MA: Allyn & Bacon, pp. 321–334.

Lee, S.W. and Kwon, J-H. (2013). The efficacy of imagery rescripting (IR) for social phobia: A randomized controlled trial. *Journal of Behavior Therapy and Experimental Psychiatry*, 44, pp. 351–360.

Morgentaler, A. (2015). *The truth about men and sex*. New York: St Martin's Griffin.

Stephens-Davidowitz, S. (2015). Searching for sex. *The New York Times*, Jan. 24.

Veale, D., Miles, S.M., Bramley, S., Muir, G. and Hodsoll, J. (2014). Am I normal? A systematic review and construction of nomograms for flaccid and erect penis length and circumference in up to 15, 521 men. *Sexual Medicine*, 115, pp. 978–986.

Veale, D., Miles, S.M., Read, J., Troglia, A., Wylie, K. and Muir, G. (2015). Sexual functioning and behavior of men with body dysmorphic disorder concerning penis size compared with men anxious about penis size and with controls: A cohort study. *Sexual Medicine*, 3, pp. 147–155.

Chapter 6

"If This Happens Again, I'll Die"

Overcoming Panic Disorder

Jess's Story

It's 9.00 am Monday morning, and I am waiting for a client that I am due to see for her first treatment session and when I meet her she is in a great deal of distress. I open the door to a tall, well-dressed young woman who is crying and shaking and being comforted by an equally tall athletic looking young man who appears to be her partner. I introduce myself, and Jess's husband Tony, as I later find him to be, helps her follow me to the therapy room. I notice how she is gripping his arm tightly with one hand whilst seeking support from the hallway wall as though she is in danger of collapsing. As we enter the therapy room Jess's breathing becomes increasingly erratic and she labours to take deep breaths as she sinks into a chair putting her face in her hands. Tony asks her if she wants him to stay and she nods. He looks at me to check that I am in agreement and I smile and gesture to a chair at the other end of the room where he seats himself and glances solicitously at Jess who seems to be regaining her composure. After a while, she looks up at me and begins speaking in shaky voice.

"Sorry about that. I knew this would be difficult, that's why I came with Tony. To be honest, I nearly turned away when we arrived but he managed to get me thorough the front door."

I smile at her and realise that I have to set a very gentle pace during our first session or risk losing her immediately. I begin softly.

"I'm really pleased that you decided not to turn around and go. I'm sure it must have been challenging for you to come here but I really think I can help you. Do you mind telling me when the problem began?"

I have had a telephone conversation with Jess prior to her referral but I want to revisit the details with her. She has been struggling with this condition for over 6 months and I'm curious to see if the problem has worsened since our telephone conversation, and if there have been any changes in her situation. Jess looks across at Tony for reassurance and begins to answer my question.

"It began just over two years ago; I'd never had a problem with this sort of thing before. I was driving down the back streets near our home with my four

DOI: 10.4324/9781003091745-7

year old daughter Lucy. We were on the way to the supermarket and I wanted to avoid the morning rush hour traffic. Suddenly this battered white van pulled out from behind and began tailgating me. It was a narrow road with speed bumps and I was being careful with Lucy in the car because she always gets upset if I drive over the bumps too quickly. I could see two guys in the van making angry gestures. The driver started flashing his headlights and tooting. Because I was distracted looking at them in the rear view mirror, I drove too close to a parked car and clipped the back of it. I pulled up sharp and they drove into the back of me. Fortunately, they weren't driving too fast but the impact and the sound of the collision gave me a shock and then Lucy started screaming. The next thing that happened is that both guys jumped out of the van and the driver started shouting racist abuse (Jess later tells me that she is from Jamaica). I started looking around to see if anyone would help us but it was a really quiet road and there was no one around. Lucy was crying and I was starting to feel really anxious and helpless when the driver started kicking my door. I suddenly had the presence of mind to lock the doors because I didn't know what they were capable of at that point. The next instant, they'd climbed back in their van, reversed and drove away down a side street. I was sitting there shaking and trying to calm Lucy down. I couldn't move and I had to call Tony and get him to drive us home. Fortunately he was on a late shift that day as I don't know what else I'd have done."

Jess pauses, takes a few breaths, and a sip of water to calm herself and then continues.

"We got home and I managed to calm Lucy down and, to be honest, I didn't feel too bad. There wasn't much damage to the car and although those guys were aggressive, I've had to deal with much worst because I work as a security guard in a night club. Anyway, the next day I decided that I'd better pull myself together and drive to the supermarket with Lucy. I wanted to regain my confidence and I didn't want it to become an issue. On the drive there everything went ok although I did avoid the road where it had happened. I managed to find a space in the supermarket car park and helped Lucy out of the car. We were walking towards the entrance when it happened. As we were about to go into the supermarket, I had a flashback to the previous day's event and I remembered how anxious and helpless I'd felt. And then I had this thought, "what if something happened to me and I couldn't protect Lucy?". I had this terrible feeling that I wouldn't be able to breath and then everything seemed unreal—my legs started shaking and my vision was blurry. I couldn't go through with it because I thought I was going to faint so I took Lucy back to the car and, after I'd managed to calm myself down, we drove home."

Jess is silent and I wonder if I can start to help her make sense of her experience this early on in the proceedings. I'm also wondering how things have been for her since the incident she described.

"Jess, thanks so much for telling me about what happened; I know it can't have been easy recounting it. How have things been since then, how would you say the problem is affecting you now?"

"I started to get worse from the outset. At first I didn't trust myself to go shopping with Lucy in case anything happened, I'd always have to have Tony accompany us. And soon I found that I couldn't take Lucy to the park on my own or any situation where it was just the two of us. Strangely, given what happened, I'm ok driving her to places, like taking her to school."

"So you always experience these symptoms when you try to take Lucy somewhere on your own?"

"It's got worst in the last few months. Now I don't feel safe going anywhere unfamiliar on my own."

"Like shops?"

"Shops particularly but even coming here."

"Can you tell me what happens in these situations Jess?"

"I don't know. I get this sense of dread that something really bad is going to happen."

"And what do you think will happen, like when you were about to meet me earlier on?"

"Like I said, I really don't know, just this awful feeling. Sorry, I'm not being much help am I?"

It seems to me that now she is calm. Jess is unable to access what she thinks and feels when she experiences these episodes. She recalls them as a huge wave of overwhelming sensations that she can't make sense of. This presents me with an initial challenge as I need to understand as clearly as possible what is going on in her mind and body and how she is interpreting her thoughts and feelings. Without this information, I could waste valuable clinical time by going off at a wrong tangent and, even worse, losing any confidence she may have in my ability to treat her. What I have to do now is take her back out of her state of calm and deliberately induce the feelings she is avoiding so desperately. My hunch is that if I can get her to experience even just the onset of her panic symptoms, she will be able to describe to me what I need to know in order to make sense of her presentation. I know that I have to proceed carefully as she's only just met me and probably doesn't have a clear understanding of what treatment will involve in spite of me having provided her with an explanation of how CBT works during our telephone conversation.

"Jess, I need you to do something for me and it's really important. If we're to work together so that I can help you overcome this problem, we have to understand as much as is possible as to what's going on when you experience these attacks. How would you feel about walking a couple of yards down the road with me?"

Jess's state of calm disappears instantly, and she looks towards Tony who has remained helpfully silent throughout the session. She looks back at me with agitation.

"I really don't want to do it."

"Let's just try to go for a little walk together while Tony waits here. I promise that if you find it too much, we can turn around and come back. Shall we try?"

Jess nods reluctantly and I stand up gesturing encouragingly towards the door. She gets to her feet and I notice that her hands have started to tremble already and she looks distinctly unsteady on her feet. I open the door to let her out, and Jess is steadying herself against the wall as she did earlier. She continues to inch her way along the corridor in this manner, and her breathing has become more laboured. It's apparent that she's trying to control it but with great difficulty. I'm not sure if she will be able to make it to the front door so I ask,

"Jess, tell me what you notice now."

She struggles to speak but manages to force out short sentences between gasps of breath.

"Difficult breathing . . . everything's blurred . . . feel like I won't be able to breath. . . . Oh Christ, I'm going to fall over!"

Jess clutches my arm, and I help her stagger back into the therapy room where she collapses into the chair for the second time that morning, puts her face between her hands, and tries to control her breathing again. I glance over at Tony and, to his credit, although he looks concerned he doesn't intervene and seems to trust that I know what I'm doing. I wait for Jess's anxiety level to decline for a few moments but not for too long as I want her to remain in a reasonable state of arousal so that she can now access her thoughts and feelings.

"Well done Jess, that was brilliant—you did really well. What I'd like to do now is to map out what seems to be going on for you on the white board. Would that be ok?"

Jess is looking very pale now but her breathing is more even and he nods.

"What was the first thing you noticed when we started to leave the room?"

"I just . . . after I got up, I felt this rushing sensation in my head and I knew that it was about to happen."

"What was about to happen?" I begin to make notes on the whiteboard as Jess recalls her experience.

"Everything becomes blurry and unreal. It's like I'm looking through thick frosted glass and then my heart starts thundering—I can't catch my breath and my legs start shaking really badly."

"Anything else?"

"No, I notice that I've been sweating but that's about it."

"And when all of this happened, what went through your mind?"

"What do you mean?"

"Sorry, let me be clearer: what was the worst thing that you thought could happen when you were in the corridor?"

"I thought that I wouldn't be able to breath."

"And if that happened?"

"I'd die . . . or I'd faint!"

"That sounds really scary. Can I just ask you, on a scale of zero to one hundred, how much did you believe that you were going to die?"

"I don't know, 60% maybe."

"And how much did you believe you would faint?"

"100%! I could feel my legs going and my head spinning."

"Thanks Jess, this is incredibly helpful—Just a few more questions. I notice that you were trying to control your breathing, am I right about that?"

"Yes, I thought if I get enough air down my lungs, I won't suffocate."

"I noticed also that you held onto the wall and before we got back into the room you'd grabbed my arm—why was that?"

"To stop me falling down."

"Is there anything else you do to try to control the symptoms?"

"No, that's it. If it gets too much I'll sit down if I can."

I stand back from the board and invite Jess to comment on the formulation of her panic attacks. She seems calmer now and contemplates what I have written and then asks me a question.

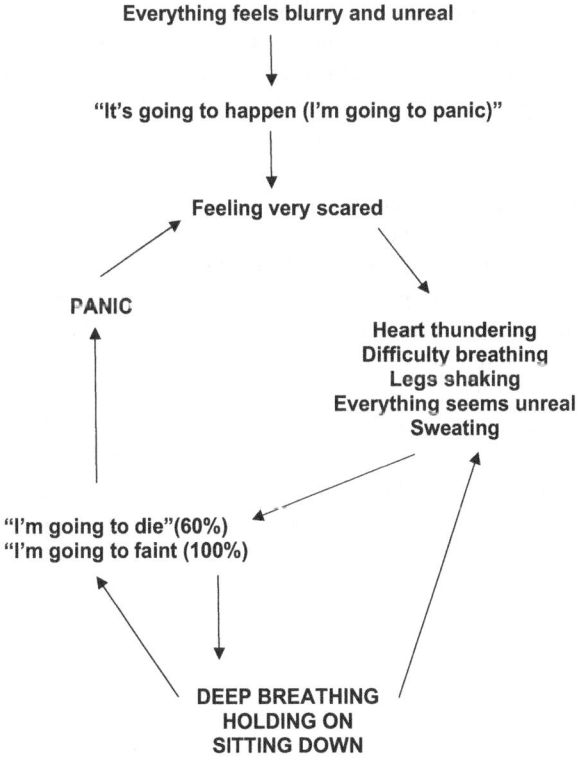

Figure 6.1 Jess's Panic Formulation

"I can see how it all fits together. I get this feeling of blurriness and I know that I'm about to have an attack. That makes me really scared and it triggers all of those physical symptoms. I'm not too sure about the direction of the arrows though. I understand that, when I get those horrible physical sensations, I'll start thinking that I'm going to die or faint and then I'll control my breathing, hold onto something or sit down. But why are the arrows going the other way, from the deep breathing to the physical sensations and to the thoughts about dying or fainting?"

"That's a really good question Jess. What do you think?"

"I really can't see the connection."

"In most cases when people experience panic attacks, they do something to reduce their feelings of anxiety. These are referred to as *safety behaviours* but they're unhelpful in two ways. Can you think of why that might be?"

"I'm sorry, I'm still not getting it."

"When you experience difficulty breathing, it's perfectly understandable that you try to control your breathing and take deeper breaths. Unfortunately what do you think happens when you *over-breathe?"*

"Is it that I get dizzy? I wondered about that?"

"Precisely, you get dizzy and everything seems unreal and blurry which leads you to believe that you're going to faint. Ironically many safety behaviours actually cause an *increase* in the initial panic symptoms rather than reducing them. But they're unhelpful in another way and keep the problem of panic attacks going in a vicious cycle. Can you see how that works?"

"Is it something to do with the arrow pointing from my safety behaviours to the thoughts about dying and fainting?"

"Exactly! You've taught yourself that when you experience these symptoms, you absolutely have to control your breathing, hold onto something or sit down. When you think back to the panic attack, you've convinced yourself that if you hadn't used these safety behaviours, you would have died or fainted. So you keep that vicious cycle going."

"So you're telling me to do nothing when this happens?"

"We're going to work together to help you overcome this problem but we have to do so in a systematic way. The first thing I have to do is teach you about what's happening in your mind and body when you have a panic attack so that you'll understand that the symptoms are uncomfortable but harmless. Do you think you can work with me on this?"

Jess confirms that she is motivated to "do what it takes" for the sake of her daughter: she wants to be able to take her shopping or to the park and feels that the panic attacks have placed constraints on the activities they previously enjoyed. Satisfied that Jess is highly motivated, we agreed a time for the next appointment and, continuing with the theme of safety behaviours, we agreed that Tony will go for a walk during our session rather than sit in the room with Jess.

At our next session, I endeavour to teach Jess about her anxiety reaction during her panic attacks, commonly known as the *fight or flight* response and explain that, although it doesn't seem to be the case, her mind and body are trying to help her but have misinterpreted the onset of the panic attack as an emergency rather than the occurrence of a benign physical symptom. She is a fast learner and I set her the task of thoroughly researching panic disorder and providing me with a mini-lecture the following week. I am using valuable clinical time to focus on what CBT therapists refer to as *psychoeducation:* providing clients with a thorough understanding of the interplay between the mental, behavioural and physical components of their disorder. This is an important foundation for us to build on but I have to lay it carefully. I will be asking Jess to drop her safety behaviours and actually invite rather than avoid a panic attack. If I haven't imparted the psychoeducation adequately, Jess will still maintain her belief that experiencing a full-blown panic attack will cause her to faint or die and refuse to engage in the next stage of treatment. I also encourage her to keep a diary recording the frequency of attacks, physical sensations, thoughts, and safety behaviours to add to our understanding.

As expected, Jess has prepared diligently and is fascinated by the intelligent design of the human mind and body to react to emergencies. She finds this topic particularly interesting in relation to her job as a nightclub security operative where she has had to deal with a number of actual *fight or flight* situations and, with her new knowledge, understands her reactions in these situations retrospectively. Jess described one such incident of a time she had to de-escalate a situation when one of the clubbers had pulled a knife on her. She told me that she remained calm and managed to contain the situation by talking to him until assistance arrived from her colleagues, and they were able to restrain him. I asked the obvious question as to why she is able to face potentially dangerous situations in her place of work on a daily basis and remain calm and yet experience panic attacks when shopping with her daughter. Jess ponders this question and explains that in the nightclub where she works, she has a much greater sense of control in any given situation. She has been trained in various protocols and procedures and relies on members of her close-knit team. Shopping with her daughter is less predictable, and she doesn't feel that she can rely on members of the public to help if anything might happen to her. This sense that something bad might happen in a completely arbitrary way has been triggered by the incident with the two men who crashed into the back of her car and verbally abused her.

"So tell me Jess, why is it virtually impossible for you to faint when you have a panic attack?"

"Because my blood pressure is really high. I'm more likely to faint when my blood pressure is low, like when I'm relaxed and I get up too quickly after I've been watching TV."

"That's great. Why's that never going to happen?"

"Because when I become really anxious, my body secretes adrenaline which make my heart pump faster and sends my blood pressure high."

"That's spot on—and why can't you suffocate in these circumstances?"

"Breathing is an automatic process and even if we tried to interfere with it, the brain would take over. I tried holding my breath for as long as I could and I really do now believe that I can't stop myself from breathing."

"What about that feeling you get that everything seems weird and unreal?"

"I found that one really interesting—*derealisation* right? So my brain's speeding up to deal with an emergency, to figure out escape routes or the moment I can attack, it just feels weird. I remember the first time I took part in a Karate tournament. When I faced my opponent I got tunnel vision, I didn't realise what it was at the time but it felt similar to derealisation. Everything in the stadium, the audience, the referee were blurred-out and all I could see was my opponent."

"It's helpful that you can link it to past experiences and that's a really good example. As we've discussed, these responses to danger have evolved over thousands of years. How was that tunnel vision helpful at the time?"

"It automatically blocked out any potential distractions and focused my attention 100% on my opponent."

"Correct. What else did you learn?"

"I think I already knew some of the more basic responses like adrenaline causing the heart to beat faster to pump blood to the major limbs like the arms and the legs to help with running or fighting and the increase in breathing to power the muscles. But I was fascinated about why people go pale in stress situations, that the body is draining blood away from the surface to the major limbs where it's most needed."

"Yes, the *peripheral circulation*. And there's another reason as to why blood drains away from the surface in a stressful situation—can you guess why?"

"I really can't think of anything other than the blood's needed elsewhere."

"It's also because if we're cut during a fight or while running away, we're less likely to bleed after our blood has drained away from the peripheral circulation."

"Amazing. I also like the bit about why we feel the need to go to the toilet when we're anxious."

"Yes, so that we're lighter if we have to run away. Helpful in an emergency but not great if you're about to give a presentation or have a job interview. So, how confident are you with your newfound knowledge that if you have a panic attack, nothing bad will happen?"

Jess pauses and thinks about this. The psychoeducation does seem to have had a positive effect as her mood seems lighter and she no longer displays the symptoms of intense anxiety that I encountered when we first met. After some moments of reflection she replies.

"I think it's definitely helped to learn this. When I feel an attack coming on I try to tell myself that it's harmless, just uncomfortable, and at one level I believe it but part of me still *feels* that it's dangerous."

Jess's response is encouraging as it indicates that, in therapeutic terms, she has developed an *intellectual understanding* of her presentation. She is able to rationalise that her symptoms are benign but when she becomes anxious, that rationality is compromised. I need to help her move on to the next stage of *emotional understanding* so that she believes in her heart as well as her head that the symptoms are benign. And the only way to help her to achieve this is through experiential learning rather than just reading around the subject and talking about it. This is where our real work begins.

"Jess, what if I could prove to you conclusively that your panic symptoms are harmless and there is no way you're going to faint or die if you drop your safety behaviours?"

"I don't know how you would be able to do that unless I had a panic attack with you in the room."

"That's precisely what I'm thinking. What we need to do is trigger the same symptoms that you experience when you have a panic attack but instead of using safety behaviours, you keep going and focus on the symptoms. I've carried this out with many clients before you and it really works."

I'm about to introduce Jess to a *hyperventilation provocation task,* part of a treatment protocol devised by Professor David Clark (Salkovskis and Clark, 1989). David Clark is something of a hero within NHS mental health services. Along with the Economist, Lord Richard Layard, he played a pivotal role in developing the Improving Access to Psychological Therapies (IAPT) serviced convincing the government to invest in the training and employment of over 6,000 new therapists within England. An overview of his work with Layard can be found in their book *Thrive* (2014). A clinical psychologist by training and now Professor of Psychology at the University of Oxford, David Clark is also renowned for developing evidence-based CBT treatment programmes particularly for panic disorder, social phobia, and PTSD, and I have been fortunate enough to attend one of his training workshops. I have also been fortunate in another way. My clinical supervisor was a member of Professor Clarke's team and has been able to impart his knowledge to me.

I map out the same simple graphs on the whiteboard that I had used with Sean and Mary in Chapter 4 to explain how Jess's avoidance of a full-blown panic attack through the use of safety behaviours is maintaining the problem and that exposure is the only way that she will learn *in her heart* that she will not faint or die during a panic attack. She asks a number of intelligent questions and then pauses, her gaze moving from the whiteboard to me. And then she says resolutely,

"OK, let's do this."

It may seem strange for medical professionals to induce the very condition that the client is seeking a cure from but, paradoxically and based on years of research, exposure to panic symptoms combined with dropping safety behaviours is the most effective method for overcoming the condition. There are a number of behavioural experiments aimed at provoking a panic attack in clients, and these are described eloquently in Professor Adrian Well's (2008) excellent book, *Cognitive Therapy of Anxiety Disorders*. One of the key principles in setting up these experiments is that the procedure triggers similar physical sensations to those that the client experiences during a panic attack. I know that Jess believes she will faint because she gets dizzy as a result of over-breathing when she becomes anxious so I have to create the same effect. If Jess had described chest pains and fear of a heart attack as many other clients do, I would have to use a procedure to bring about those particular symptoms. The other component I have to build into the experiment is what is described in clinical literature as a *disconfirmatory manoeuvre:* getting Jess to do something when her panic symptoms are at their peak to prove to her conclusively that she will not faint, no matter how dizzy she feels. I have calculated that the best approach I can use will be a *hyperventilation provocation task*. This is quite a hard-core approach as it involves both the clinician and the client deliberately hyperventilating whilst standing in front of one another and is widely used in treating panic. The reason for the method's frequent use is that it triggers a wide range of symptoms commonly experienced during panic attacks including dizziness, blurred vision, increased heart rate, breathlessness, dissociation, and feeling hot and faint. It's not a pleasant experience for the client or the therapist modelling the procedure but it is a powerful and rapid method for curing someone of panic disorder.

Hyperventilation provocation is a safe procedure and the unpleasant physical symptoms subside over the course of the exposure (van den Hout et al., 1990). However, there are four exclusion criteria for carrying out this exercise with a client: pregnancy, asthma, heart problems, and high blood pressure. I have been diagnosed with hypertension 2 years ago and have been taking medication to keep it under control. I feel some trepidation at the prospect of modelling hyperventilating for Jess but I know this is a very important moment in her treatment and, if she goes through with it, it could be a turning point in her recovery. I just hope I don't have stroke whilst doing it—that would really traumatise her. I stand up, loosen my collar, and ask her to stand up with me.

"OK Jess, I'm going to demonstrate and we're both going to continue to breathe deeply and rapidly. But just before we do, on a scale of zero to one hundred, how much do you believe you will die if you had a full-blown panic attack?"

"Having learned everything we've covered about the fight or flight response, I no longer believe that I will die. But in spite of what I've learned, I still *feel* as though I will probably faint. I'd rate that as 60%."

I am encouraged by Jess's response which indicates that the psychoeducation has had some impact. She no longer believes that she will die, and her belief that she will faint has reduced by 40% from our first session. I note this prediction on the whiteboard. I turn to her.

"OK Jess, start breathing with me!"

I begin to breathe rapidly and loudly making encouraging gestures with my hands for Jess to follow. She begins hesitantly but forces herself to breathe in and out faster until we are both gasping and panting at one another. At times like these I find myself wondering what someone passing by in the corridor might think of the sounds emanating from the therapy room. Even my verbal encouragement might sound dubious:

"Keep going, don't stop—faster!"

But these momentary thoughts disappear as I feel myself becoming increasingly dizzy, and I know that Jess is feeling this too as she has become quite pale and is staggering slightly. Between gasps I ask her,

"How much do you believe you're going to faint?"

"80!"

"Keep going, you're doing really well."

To her credit, Jess forces herself to breathe in and out even faster and tears have started to run down her cheeks. At the same time, I can feel veins bulging in my forehead and have a metallic taste in my mouth. I'm feeling slightly nauseous and my brain is full of fog, vision blurring slightly. I notice that Jess is attempting to steady herself against the wall.

"No Jess, don't do that. Watch me. Stand on one leg—try!"

I manage to balance on one leg somewhat shakily and wobble about in an ungainly fashion but manage to stay upright. Jess gamely follows my lead in spite of her tears, continuing to inhale and exhale raggedly whilst maintaining a trembling one-legged stance.

"Brilliant Jess. Now watch me and try this."

I spin round clockwise inducing further dizziness and tottering about in front of her like a drunk. She has stopped crying and actually laughs at my undignified cavorting. She follows suit and we totter around the room like inebriated dervishes.

"Now stand on one leg again."

Once more we both manage to strike an unsteady pose burdened by the fog of our dizziness, but I sense a lightening in her anxiety. Jess has pushed herself to the point where she is beginning to realise that she will not faint no matter how dizzy and physically awful she feels right now.

"Now how much do you believe you'll faint?" She gasps out an answer:

"30!"

We're home and dry. We remain standing and I track her belief ratings on the whiteboard for another 5 minutes until she reaches 10% and I ask her to sit down. We both collapse in our chairs, and I congratulate myself for not having a stroke. I also congratulate Jess on the courage she has shown by throwing herself into the experiment with such vigour in spite of her anxiety. I ask her how she is feeling and she grins at me which is encouraging.

"Like shit, I've got a headache."

"So have I but don't worry, it'll subside. I know it was very challenging and well done for seeing it through, but what did you learn from it?"

"I really thought I was going to faint at one point and couldn't believe that I was able to stand on one leg. My head still feels foggy but I guess I've learned that I *probably* wouldn't faint as that's the worst panic attack I've experienced—I normally do something to stop things getting that bad." Jess pauses and I probe her as to her remaining doubt. She takes a sip of water before she replies.

"It's one thing doing this in a therapy room with you on hand. Part of me was thinking that if I *did* faint, you'd take care of me—that helped me to follow through. But it's another thing for me to take a chance on taking Lucy to a supermarket. If I did faint, I really don't think anyone would help me and I'd worry about what would happen to her."

"So how do you think we can solve this problem?"

"I've no idea. There's no way I'd carry out any sort of experiment on me going into a supermarket with Lucy and I don't think I'd even chance going to one on my own."

A plan is beginning to form in my mind but I feel the need to suggest it very tentatively as we are making good progress and I don't want to push Jess too far too quickly.

"How would it be if we visited a supermarket together? Do you trust me?"

"What do you mean, get me to have a panic attack in the middle of a supermarket, you must be joking!"

"No, nothing so extreme. What I'm suggesting is that we do just what I've said: visit the supermarket together and see what happens, just walk around the place."

"I can't say I find the thought that appealing but I feel as though I've made a lot of progress today so I'm willing to try it out. But if we get there and I don't want to go through with it, I reserve the right to pull out."

I agree to Jess's terms and we arrange to meet the following week. Jess's confidence has grown to the extent that she is able to drive to our sessions unaccompanied which is helpful so we agree to take her car to the supermarket.

The following week the weather is ominously overcast and rain lashes down outside as I dash out to meet Jess having received a text message informing me that she has just arrived. I am not relishing the prospect of our next behavioural experiment as, yet again, it will involve me going outside of my own comfort zone and I am starting to feel gloomy and slightly on edge about the number of things that might go wrong. Then I remember a very helpful CBT principle that I often bang on about to my clients and remind myself that I need to follow my own advice. *Emotional reasoning* means interpreting what's happening to you through the lens of your emotions. If we feel low and anxious for whatever reason, we're more likely to see negative aspects within the situation or threats that might not exist and this, in turn, often affects the way we act. Right now I'm feeling cold and slightly despondent but I can't afford to anticipate the outcome of our behavioural experiment through the lens of my negative emotions. I also remind myself of the psychologist E. A. Holmes (Holmes, Lang and Shah, 2009) and colleagues' findings that imagining a positive outcome when goal setting will increase the chances of you achieving your objective. I resolve to pull myself together and focus on what I have to do. Jess leans over and opens the passenger door of a very new 4 × 4 BMW, way above my paygrade. It is immaculate and fragrant inside. The heater is on and already my spirits are lifting.

As we drive to the supermarket through gloomy suburban streets lurching over speed bumps I think of the example my clinical supervisor has set me in carrying out behavioural experiments and his apparent fearlessness in challenging himself. A couple of years ago we were both attending a one-day workshop on using behavioural experiments in CBT delivered by a highly talented therapist from the Oxford Cognitive Therapy Centre by the name of Dr. Martina Mueller. After a morning of theory, Martina used the afternoon to challenge us with some experiential learning. Our brief was to carry out a personal behavioural experiment within the grounds or the vicinity of the training venue and report back in two hours. I was sitting next to my supervisor and wanted to impress him in a rather childish way so I thought I'd try an experiment that was a little less mundane than the examples that I'd heard discussed around me (e.g. going to the canteen and deliberately complaining about a cup of coffee at the front of the queue). I borrowed a stick of lipstick from a colleague, went into the toilet, and proceeded to apply it to my face until I'd transformed my complexion into a garish shade of crimson. I'd read about this type of behavioural experiment in the case of a therapist treating a client for social phobia with a fear of blushing. The client's phobia had become so entrenched that he avoided being served in shops for fear that he would be judged and draw a negative response from staff. In order to test this prediction, the therapist had liberally applied blusher and visited a number of shops with the client without receiving any adverse reaction. Eager to impress I came back from the toilet and presented myself to my supervisor who told me to apply even more lipstick until I looked as though I had some kind of rabid skin infection. He then thought it would be a good idea to take me and another colleague on a tour of the campus parading me with my bizarre appearance and randomly talking to Police Officers, security staff, and complete strangers. My colleague began to look uneasy when my supervisor took me into a rough-looking youth club, interrupted a game of pool, and asked what was going on there. Fortunately, we met with a friendly response. The grand finale was when we entered a tube station and he told one of the guards that I was his client and suffering from claustrophobia. Would it be ok if we visited the platform? The experiment was taking on a life of its own as the guard accompanied us down the escalator and onto the platform and my supervisor seemed elated at how far he could push boundaries. It was at this point that a train thundered through the tunnel and pulled to a stop with the driver's cabin next to us. He then took it upon himself to ask the driver to stop the train so that I could wander about the carriage in front of the passengers for a few moments. We must have looked like a weird entourage to the commuters (they probably thought we would start busking) but no one paid us any attention and we left the station after thanking the driver and the guard.

On reflection, the value of the experience was less about testing predictions concerning the public's response to my bizarre appearance (there wasn't any). It was more an exercise in Albert Ellis (2004) inspired *shame attacking* that we encountered with Martin in Chapter 6. My own experience of "shame attacking" during the workshop 2 years ago was to stand me in good stead as we pulled into the Tesco's car park. I turn to Jess and outline my plan.

"So, we're going to go into the supermarket, walk around for a while. Then I'm going to purchase something so we'll queue up at the till and leave. Now, how likely do you think it is that you'll have a panic attack?"

"I feel nervous but after what we did last week and with you accompanying me, I don't think I'll have a panic attack. But the problem is that I'm still scared of having a panic attack when I'm on my own, or even worse, when I'm with Lucy."

"And what's the worst thing about having a panic attack even if you were with Lucy? You know that you won't suffocate and you definitely won't faint, so what is it?"

"I know that but I just don't think anyone would help. I'd also feel really bad, stupid."

"Why?"

"Because of what people would think of me."

"How would you know that they were thinking badly of you?"

"I don't know, they'd laugh or say something nasty."

"You really believe that?"

"Yes."

As I'd expected, Jess's catastrophic beliefs about suffocating or fainting have declined after last week's experiment but she is still stuck with her secondary negative belief that if she experiences some sort of distress in public other people will ignore her, or worse, openly mock her. In order to set up the experiment so that she will learn from it, I have to determine the strength of her beliefs.

"So, on a scale of zero to one hundred, how much do you believe that people would ignore you and your daughter if you had a panic attack?"

"I reckon 90%"

"And what about the possibility of them laughing or saying something nasty?"

"That's a bit lower, probably 50%"

"OK, this is how we're going to test those beliefs. We're going to go into the store and after your anxiety has declined to a level we're both happy with, we'll queue up at the checkout and I'll pretend to faint."

"You'll do what? Are you crazy?"

"No, I'm completely serious—are you up for this?"

For the second time in our work together, Jess starts to laugh and I get the sense that her desire to see me make a prat of myself is stronger than her anxiety about entering the store. As we leave the car and walk towards the entrance, I can feel a spike of adrenaline and my heart starts beating faster. I'm hoping that my predictions about human altruism amongst the shopping public are correct today and try not to let my mind focus on potential negative outcomes, like being restrained by a store detective for example.

We walk into the harsh neon lighting of the store, and I notice that it is very busy at this time of day. That's helpful as it will increase Jess's stress level, and I can tell that she is already beginning to feel anxious by the expression on her face. As we walk down the dairy aisle I turn to her.

"What's your anxiety rating now?"

"80%"

"What would increase it?"

"Going down a busier aisle."

"Ok, go towards the anxiety. It's your best chance of overcoming it."

Jess gamely marches to the bakery aisle and is jostled by several elderly shoppers loading cakes into their trollies. I maintain a distance so that there isn't any chance of Jess obtaining reassurance from my presence near her. We proceed in this manner for around 15 minutes, and I frequently check her anxiety rating until it has declined to a gratifying 10%. I am confident that Jess has learned that she is now able to visit a supermarket unaccompanied without the risk of experiencing a panic attack. Mindful of the time and my other scheduled appointments, I grit my teeth and accept that the moment has come to lead by example. I have selected a packet of sandwiches, drink, and item of fruit as part of a "meal deal" and lead Jess to the check-out. She has a basket with several grocery items. As we queue I am evaluating the shoppers in front of and behind us. They seem to be representative of the average cross-section of shoppers you might find in any outer London supermarket on any day of the week and I am reassured that none of them has an outwardly aggressive demeanour. The middle aged couple in front of me have paid for their shopping and are finishing off packing. Jess is watching me expectantly as I place my items in front of the woman behind the till. I can feel myself hesitating so I force myself to take a deep breath and then slide to the floor clutching the side of the counter and groaning. I slump onto my backside and raise a trembling hand to my forehead. The anxiety I am feeling at making a display of myself is actually making my act of having a panic attack more convincing. I look up and am surrounded by concerned, attentive faces looking down at me. A member of staff kneels down and places a solicitous hand on my arm.

"Are you ok sir?"

I am feeling a little guilty now as she looks genuinely concerned but I notice Jess observing this exchange intently and feel vindicated. If this minor inconvenience to the staff and customers is the price for curing Jess of her fears, it's worth paying. I reply slowly.

"I'm really sorry, this sometimes happens to me when I queue up in supermarkets. Don't worry, I just need a moment."

"It's no problem. Take all the time you want. I'll just fetch a first-aider."

I didn't foresee that consequence and need to find a way of extricating myself from the situation. I don't want to put the staff to any further inconvenience or invite the interest of a store detective who might think this is an elaborate scam to avoid paying for my "meal deal." I gently decline her offer and slowly get to my feet clutching the counter for support. I turn to look at the other shoppers and say bashfully,

"I'm really sorry, I feel so embarrassed."

I burly, heavily tattooed gentleman steps forward and pats me on the shoulder reassuringly.

"Listen mate, don't worry about it. I've had panic attacks in the past so I know how you feel. You've nothing to be ashamed of."

The other shoppers are smiling encouragingly, and I feel humbled by his and their kindness towards me. I try to counter my guilty thoughts with my previous justification about supporting Jess's recovery and also the realisation that the staff and shoppers feel good about their altruism. I thank everyone profusely, pay for my lunch, and walk out of the store closely followed by Jess. We get into her car for a debriefing to avoid further scrutiny. She is beaming at me and says,

"You must do some crazy shit in your job!"

"Quite. But what do you think now? On a scale of zero to one hundred, how much do you believe that people would ignore you and your daughter if you had a panic attack?"

"After seeing that, zero definitely. Everyone was so kind to you, I couldn't believe it. Especially that bloke who confessed to having panic attacks in front of a bunch of strangers."

"And what about the possibility of people laughing or saying something nasty if you had a panic attack?"

"I'd say there's always a slight possibility but now it feels like 5% after the way those people reacted."

"That's great. Now, can you give me a lift back?"

As Jess drives us back, I can feel a slight tension headache following the rush of adrenaline and feel slightly queasy every time we go over a speed bump as she takes a shortcut down the back streets to avoid heavy traffic on the main road. Suddenly she stops the car on a narrow road of terraced houses looking out onto a nondescript green. I ask her why she has stopped here.

"This is where it happened, where those guys tailgated me and I had my first panic attack with Lucy in the car. I've been avoiding this route since it happened but after the supermarket today I wanted to come back. It feels as though, with your help, I've beaten it and I can get my life back on track."

"We've still got another four sessions. We can set up some more experiments so that you feel really confident in your recovery."

"If it's ok with you, I'd rather end today. Going into that supermarket with you was the best thing I could have done. I really know in my heart that there's no way I'm going to faint and you've restored my trust in the public. I'm going to take Lucy shopping tomorrow."

I feel a little uncomfortable ending therapy with Jess so abruptly as I usually complete a relapse prevention plan with each client to raise awareness of any problems recurring and contingency plans for dealing with them. However, she is resigned to her course of action and as she drops me off we agree that I will contact her in 3 months to check that she has made a full recovery. She is about to drive off but winds down her window and calls out to me.

"How many times have you done that?"

"What?"

"Fainted in a supermarket like that?"

"My first time."

She drives away laughing and I wave her off with just enough time to eat my "meal deal" before the next client.

References

Clark, D.M. (1986). A cognitive model of panic. *Behaviour Research and Therapy*, 24, pp. 461–470.

Clark, D.M. (1989). Anxiety states: Panic and generalised anxiety. In: K. Hawthorn, P.M. Salkovskis, Joan Kirk and D.M. Clark, eds., *Cognitive behaviour therapy for psychiatric problems a practical guide*. Oxford: Oxford University Press.

Ellis, A. (2004) The road to tolerance. In: *The philosophy of rational emotive behaviour therapy*. New York. Prometheus Books.

Holmes, E.A., Lang T.J. and Shah, D.M. (2009). Developing interpretation bias modification as a 'cognitive vaccine' for depressed mood: Imagining positive events makes you feel better than thinking about them verbally. *Journal of Abnormal Psychology*, 118, pp. 76–88.

Layard, R. and Clark, D.M. (2014). *Thrive: The power of evidence-based psychological therapies*. London: Penguin.

Salkovskis, J.K. and Clark, D.M., eds. (1989). *Cognitive behaviour therapy for psychiatric problems. A practical guide.* Oxford: Oxford University Press.

Van den Hout, M.A., de Jong, P., Zanderberger, J. and Merckelbach, H. (1990). Waning of panic sensations during prolonged hyperventilation. *Behaviour Research and Therapy,* 28, pp. 445–448.

Wells, A. (2008). *Cognitive therapy of anxiety disorders—a practice manual and conceptual guide.* Chichester: Wiley.

Chapter 7

"It Isn't in My Head"

Vomit Phobia and Fear of Soiling

Mary's Story

Mary is sitting opposite me at our first session together, and I am struck by how pale her complexion is along with dark rings beneath her slightly bulging eyes. Every time Mary speaks her breath smells incredibly sour even though there is some distance between us. I feel uncharitable about this last observation as she has, on first impressions, a warm, friendly personality in spite of her apparent anxiety at attending our first session. Mary explains that for years she has had a fear of being sick in public and this has significantly constrained her life. She tells me that she had a successful career as a PR manager until one day.

"I was due to give a presentation to the senior management team on our latest strategy and I remember feeling unusually queasy half an hour before the meeting. I was used to public speaking as part of my job and could normally manage my "butterflies" before a presentation but this was different. Up until then I'd always felt anxiety as a tingling sensation in my stomach that I could override and on most occasions, once I started speaking the feelings would go away because I wasn't paying them any attention. But on that day I felt this heavy, nauseous feeling that kept growing and I became convinced that I would throw up during the presentation. Ten minutes before the meeting I approached my boss and told her that I was feeling really ill and had to go home. Everyone was very sympathetic on that occasion and I tried to ignore it as an isolated incident. I noticed that the feelings of nausea went away as soon as I'd left the building. But then things got worse."

"In what way?"

"Soon I'd get these feelings of nausea when I attended meetings, even if I didn't have to present. Before long it became difficult for me to even meet with people one-to-one without starting to feel sick and I'd often make excuses to leave."

"How did you cope?"

DOI: 10.4324/9781003091745-8

"Not very well. The only thing I could do was avoid breakfast and lunch. I'd lost my appetite anyway when I was in work. The one thing that comforted me were cigarette breaks and I know it's not healthy, but I started to smoke more. The only thing that just about got me through meetings was that I constantly sipped water."

I look down at the side of her chair and notice that Mary has a large bottle of still mineral water next to her. As if my glance has drawn her attention to it, she picks up the bottle and takes a series of gulps. She continues.

"Every time I felt the nausea rising, I would take a few sips. I figured that it would "flush it back down" and prevent me from being sick."

"And did it?"

"Yes, but only temporarily. The problem was getting worse and worse. I was making all sorts of excuses to get out of presentations and meetings. My boss was showing signs of concern but I was too embarrassed to tell her about my problem. Eventually I knew that I couldn't carry on anymore and I agreed with my boss to change my role in the company for a far less responsible position. That was a year ago and I've worked from home since then."

"I'm really sorry to hear that. What's going on in your life at the moment?"

Mary stares at the table between us and becomes tearful. I offer her a tissue, and she drinks from her bottle before regaining her composure.

"There's not much going on at all. I've moved in with my sister because I couldn't afford to pay the rent on my flat. I used to have a nice apartment and a company car but that's a distant memory. The problem's got worse over the past few years and it's dominating my life. I hardly go anywhere for fear of being sick. Friends have drifted away because I haven't kept in touch and I couldn't bring myself to tell them the reason—only my family know."

"How did you manage to get here today?"

"My sister lives near here so I walked, that was OK. I got here just before the time of the appointment and I checked where the toilet was."

"I see. You seem to be managing ok right now though."

"It's because you're a medical professional—if I threw up in front of you it wouldn't be so bad. I don't think you'd judge me negatively."

"What's brought you to therapy now?"

"I'm sick of living my life like this. The only thing I can manage to do is go to the local shops in the evening when hardly anyone is around. I turned 35 this year and I thought, I've got to do something about this otherwise my whole life will be wasted. Do you think you can help me?"

I pause for a moment before I answer. Mary has described classic symptoms of what is labelled in clinical literature as "specific phobia of vomiting" or *emetophobia* (Emesis is the Greek word for the act of vomiting), and this condition is considered by many clinicians as challenging and difficult to treat

(Veale and Lambrou, 2006). This is because clients frequently drop out or don't respond to treatment. The Diagnostic and Statistical Manual of Mental Disorders—DSM-5 (2013) is considered to be the "psychiatrist's bible" worldwide for diagnosing psychological presentations but merely lists emetophobia as "Specific Phobias—other." Boschen (2007) notes that this ambiguous label has had the unfortunate result that the condition has had the effect of attracting very little interest (and funding) from researchers. In some ways, emetophobia is similar to the panic phobia we encountered with Jess in Chapter 6 but differs in that people with this condition are thought to have a chronic fear of losing control (Davidson, Boyle and Lauchlan, 2008) that maintains the problem. Given these facts, I am a little tentative with my reply and answer Mary's question with a question.

"How committed are you to working on this problem?"

"I have to make it work. I can't go on living like this."

"The first thing I need you to do is complete a detailed diary for me over the next week, hour by hour describing what situations you're in, what you're thinking and how you're feeling. It's vitally important for our work together because we both need to understand how your problem came about and what's keeping it going. Can you do that for me?"

Mary nods. I provide her with the diary pro forma and we schedule our next appointment together.

When we meet the following week, I am dismayed that Mary's diary reveals very little that will further our mutual understanding of her problem. She wasn't exaggerating when she said that there wasn't much going on in her life. Her notes reveal a crushingly monotonous daily routine of getting up late, carrying out her work duties remotely, watching TV and surfing the internet with occasional trips to the local shops late in the evening. My additional disappointment is that none of the activities that Mary has engaged in over the past week have triggered any vomit-phobic responses that we could dissect to obtain a better understanding of her condition. From what she has recorded, Mary seems to experience a constant feeling of low-level nausea but avoids any situation in which she would not be able to escape swiftly if her nausea and perceived risk of vomiting were to increase. I put this dilemma to her, and she looks despondent so I ask her a question as a plan begins to form in my mind.

"Can you remember the last time you really thought that you would vomit in public?"

"It was couple of weeks ago. I was in mini-supermarket late at night and there wasn't anyone there when I went in. But when I went to pay, a few people had come into the shop and I had to queue. I started to feel sick and I left without buying anything."

"What was going through your mind when that happened?"

"I can't remember. All I can tell you is that I felt sick and knew I had to get out of there."

"The problem we have Mary, is that unless we know exactly what's going on for you in these situations it'll be difficult to know how to proceed. I have an idea. How would you feel if we both went across the road and paid a visit to the mini-market?"

Mary blanches at my suggestion and her body stiffens.

"I really don't want to do that."

"Look Mary, I'm not going to do anything without your consent and you can turn back if things become too intense for you. We'll just walk across to the shop and I want you to tell me everything that you're thinking and feeling ok?"

Mary looks very unhappy at the prospect of this but nods, puts on her coat, and picks up her bottle of water. She immediately takes a few gulps and we set off. It's yet another grim, overcast day and the meagre parade of shops look uninviting but they have stood me in constant good stead on occasions such as this. I can feel a biting December wind and realise that in my enthusiasm to get Mary to engage in the experiment before she changes her mind, I have neglected to put my jacket on. However, my discomfort is rewarded as Mary provides me with a running commentary as we cross the road.

"I can feel my stomach churning now and it's getting worse. It feels as though it's rising up in my throat." She opens her bottle of water and takes several gulps.

"I know that if I go in that shop I'll be sick. It's getting worse."

"Are there any images that come up for you?"

"I don't want to talk about it . . . I want to go back now please."

Mary is leaning against the window of the shop and looks even more ashen-faced than usual. I congratulate her on making such a positive effort, and we return to the warmth of the room both relieved in our own ways. When we get back to our room, Mary takes a seat but I go over to the whiteboard intent on capturing her perception of the experience whilst it is fresh in her mind.

"Thanks so much for going through with that Mary, I know it was challenging for you but you did really well. Thinking back on it, what was the first thing you noticed that changed as we were leaving?"

"I noticed that my stomach lurched and the sick feeling started to spread up my throat." I start to make notes on the whiteboard.

"It sounds as though you're constantly alert for feelings of increased nausea—am I right?"

"Now you put it like that, yes, I'm always aware of the feeling. It's always there at some level."

"And when you noticed that feeling of nausea increase, what did you think?"

"I thought, if we go into that shop I'm definitely going to be sick."

"And when you had that thought, how did you feel?"

"Even worse, I could feel it rising."

"I noticed that you started drinking water outside the shop, why was that?"

"To prevent me from being sick, to force it back down again."

"And did it help?"

"Just a little bit."

"And what would the worst thing be if you were sick Mary?"

"It would be horrible, I don't think I could stand the feeling."

"Why, do you think it would be dangerous, that you would choke or something?"

"No, not that. I just think it would feel horrible."

"Is there anything else that would be bad about being sick in the street or the shop.?"

"People would see me, I'd hate that."

"Why?"

"Because they'd think I'm some drunk or a druggie scumbag?"

"How do you know they'd think that?"

"They'd shout at me."

"What you're describing sounds really vivid. Do you get any images when this happens, when it happened earlier?"

"I can see me projectile vomiting with bulging eyes, other people looking at me with disgust."

"It sounds to me as though the fear of being judged by other people worries you more than the physical act of vomiting, have I got that right?"

"Yes, but I'd still hate it. I think it would go on and on and feel awful."

"When's the last time you vomited?" Mary pauses and reflects on the question. She sips her water and then replies.

"I don't think I've been sick since I was seven years of age. But I can remember that occasion as though it was last week. My parents had enrolled me in a Judo class because I was getting bullied at school and I was due to attend the first lesson. My mum thought it would be a good idea to give me a big, cooked lunch so that I would have plenty of energy for the class. I remember feeling very nervous when I joined the class with the other girls. I was wearing a stiff new Judo outfit and felt very self-conscious. We started doing various exercise including break-falls on the mat and I began to feel queasy. The feeling got worse and worse as the class went on and then we had to do partner work on the mat, a bit like wrestling. I was paired up with this older girl and she was being quite rough with me. She turned me over violently so that I was on top of her and at that moment it all came out, I was sick all over her. I can see her look of anger and disgust and all of the other girls laughing at me. I ran off the mat into the changing room and never went back."

Mary's description of this event has been so vivid that it feels as though I am there witnessing this poor little girl's humiliation. I put my pen down and sit opposite her as she is looking at the floor and I feel the need to re-connect with her.

"Does that memory come up for you very often Mary?"

"I think I managed to block it out for years but after the incident at work with the presentation, it's come up quite often, sometimes just fleetingly."

"Did it come up just now, when we were visiting the shops?"

Mary nods despondently, and I make my final notes on the whiteboard. I draw her attention to the simple formulation I have mapped out as a starting point to helping us develop a shared understanding of her problem and to check whether my assumptions are correct from her perspective.

"I'm trying to make sense of what's going on for you and what's keeping the problem going. What do you make of this?"

Mary considers the formulation for a few moments before replying.

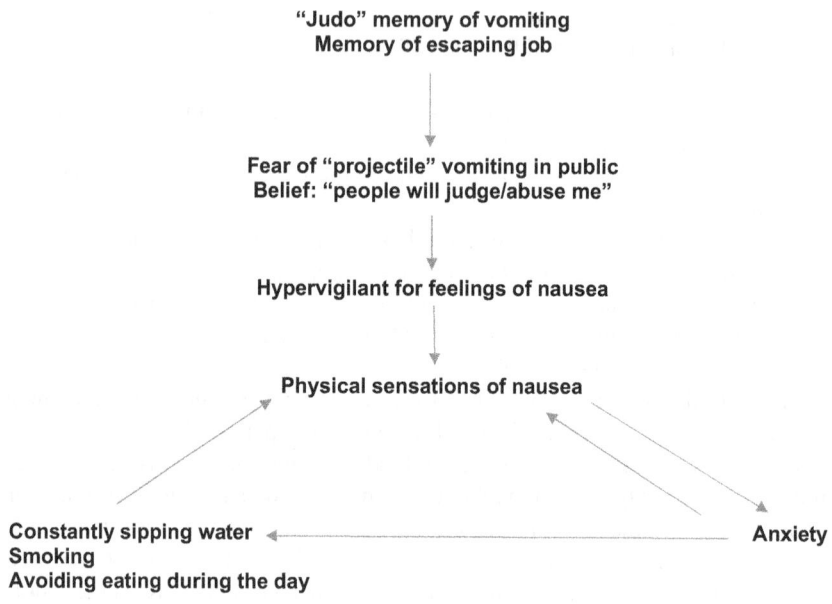

Figure 7.1 Formulation of Mary's Fear of Vomiting

"I hadn't thought of it like that before. I think you're right—those memories are a big part of it but what do you mean by hypervigilant for feelings of nausea?"

"From what you've said it sounds as though you're constantly scanning your stomach for the slightest hint of nausea. Perhaps you don't even know you're doing it most of the time but because it's such a threat, your mind is on guard even below your level of awareness."

"That makes sense, the way you describe it. I think I am constantly on guard and the only time I can really switch off is when I feel safe at home. I'm not sure about the rest of it—the triangle at the bottom?"-

"If you're constantly scanning for feelings of nausea, what's likely to happen?"

"I'm bound to notice something."

"And when you notice something, how do you feel?"

"Anxious."

"People experience feelings of anxiety in different ways. Some notice a tightness in their chest or increased heart-beat: where do you notice it?"

"In my stomach."

"So you get that vicious cycle: the feeling of nausea triggers anxiety and the anxiety in turn causes you to feel increasingly nauseous."

"What about the rest of it? I can see that I sip water because I get anxious about being sick but are you saying it increases the feeling of nausea?"

"Think about it. You restrict eating until the evening so you have nothing in your stomach. If you keep sipping water all day and smoking on an empty stomach, it's not surprising that you feel queasy. Also, the more frequently you sip water, what are you focusing on?"

"The possibility that I might be sick?"

"Absolutely. You're increasing your preoccupation with sensations in your stomach." I notice that our time is nearly up but am encouraged when Mary asks if she can take a photo of the formulation on her mobile.

"Please do and try to compare any incidents throughout the week with the diagram we've come up with. Also, please keep the diary going but try to be aware of the subtle details that we've noticed today hour-by-hour."

After Mary has left I ponder on how best to proceed. I have re-visited Professor David Veale's (2009) helpful protocol on using a CBT approach to treat "specific phobia of vomiting" and am considering how to adapt this to her specific presentation. She does not seem anxious about the prospect of seeing other people vomiting which is common with this presentation and something I have encountered before. That part of treatment is easier to set up as it involves simple exposure methods similar to those used with other phobias. I have a number of helpful photos stored on my laptop that I have used previously for this purpose including favourites such as "man retching," "pavement vomit," and "pigeons and vomit." The protocol also involves exposure to fake vomit: tinned vegetable soup is a favourite with added Butyric acid for that authentic "vomity" smell. I decide to follow Professor Veale's recommended starting point and focus on psychoeducation, determining how much Mary knows about the act of vomiting and trying to normalise it as a helpful bodily function.

When we meet the following week, I am encouraged by the fact that Mary's diary captures far more subtle detail than her previous attempt. It transpires that she occasionally goes for walks with her sister along the banks of a nearby river even in the middle of Winter when weather permits. It would appear from her entries that Mary is almost oblivious to feelings of nausea on these occasions and has no fear of vomiting. I ask her what she makes of this.

"I guess it's what you mentioned last week, I'm not, what's the word you used, *hypervigilant* for any feelings in my stomach. It feels like such a rare escape from my sister's house when the weather's OK and she can come with me, that I really enjoy every moment."

"And what's missing on those occasions?"

"Other people."

"That's absolutely right. There's no threat, no possibility that you'll be sick in front of other people and draw their disgust. So what do you make of this insight?"

"That I need to avoid other people."

"You could spend the rest of your life doing that but you told me that you wanted to get your life back so that's not really possible is it? It seems to me that you believe that you're more physically pre-disposed to vomiting than most people, have I got that right?"

"Yes."

"So why do the feelings of nausea go away when no one is around?"

"Because I'm not anxious?"

"Exactly. So that's telling us that you're no more likely to vomit than anyone else and that it's an anxiety problem rather than a physical condition."

I use Mary's insight as an opportunity to enthuse us about the many benefits that nature has bestowed upon us by providing us with a vomit reflex. It helps with our survival when we are ill. It prevents us from contracting various diseases by ridding us of toxins. Top tip: rats are the only animals on the planet who are unable to vomit which is why they are doomed to expire after eating rat poison (I borrowed this from the Veale paper). In spite of my best efforts, Mary remains nonplussed.

"It may be a helpful 'mechanism' as you call it but I still think it looks disgusting and other people will find it disgusting."

"If you saw someone vomiting in public, what would you think?"

"That they were drunk or on drugs."

"But what other reason could there be?"

"I suppose they might be ill."

It had briefly occurred to me to ask Mary to conduct a survey amongst her friends posing the question: "If you saw someone being sick in public, what would you think?" but remember that she has lost contact with most of them. This is a very popular method amongst CBT therapists for a variety of psychological presentations and is aimed at challenging clients' negative predictions about how other people will act or think. I've always been sceptical about this approach and when I've tried it, there has been very little shift in the client's beliefs. This is probably because they have inferred that people responding to the survey are unrepresentative of the general public. I have already decided that a more radical behavioural experiment is necessary and have purchased a tub of vegetable soup for the purpose (without the Butyric acid on this occasion).

"Yes Mary, that's what people might think. Let's suppose for a moment that I was sick in the street in front of people, how do you think they would react?"

"I think they'd say something and probably look disgusted."

"On a scale of zero to one hundred, how much do you believe that?"

"90%"

"And what would 'looking disgusted' look like, could you show me?" Mary grimaces twisting her features into a caricature of repugnance.

"So we're going to put your theory to the test. We'll walk over the road to that parade of shops and I'll pretend to be sick in a very convincing way and I want you to watch closely how people nearby react."

Mary is visibly taken aback by my suggestion and looks incredulous.

"Are you *really* going to do that?"

"I'm completely serious. Wait here and I'll fetch my jacket."

I have planned this the previous evening, and I quickly retrieve my tub of fresh vegetable soup from the fridge and quickly slop some of the content into a small sealable plastic bag that I tuck carefully into my inside jacket pocket. As I collect Mary and we leave the room, I feel the familiar rush of nerves in anticipation of carrying out this particular experiment. The neighbourhood in the immediate vicinity isn't particularly genteel and I hope this doesn't result in me getting punched which would confirm Mary's negative belief. It's one thing pretending to faint in a supermarket as I did with Jess but throwing up in the high street might attract a less charitable response. However, I'm willing to risk it as I can't think of another way to disconfirm Mary's belief as there's no way that she would try this out.

We cross the road and follow the curve of the parade of shops and I can see a cluster of people standing outside the bakers, mothers with small children and a couple of workmen eating sausage rolls—perhaps not the ideal audience but time is running out for our session. I reach into my jacket pocket, turn away, and surreptitiously swig the cold soup suppressing a slight feeling of disgust. As I approach the group, I check that Mary is close by, observing my actions. It seems that her fascination with the unfolding event has momentarily reduced her anxiety of being around other people. I notice a litter bin near the group and totter towards it feigning illness. I then lean over the bin and expel the cold vegetable soup accompanied by loud retching sounds and dramatic convulsions. I pause for a moment, look up towards the group with a contrite expression, apologise briefly, and walk on unsteadily.

We make it back to the room and I mop my chin with a tissue, Mary is regarding me with a bemused expression. When we are seated I ask her to tell me exactly what she observed.

"Well, they just looked at you, a bit surprised, like no big deal. The blokes kept on eating and the women carried on talking."

"Any evident disgust like you predicted?" I pull a face imitating Mary's rictus expression before we had left the clinic. She laughs for the first time we have been working together.

"No, nothing I could see."

"So, if *you* were sick in the street in front of people, on a scale of zero to one hundred, how much do you believe they would react with <u>visible</u> disgust?"

"OK, less than 90 but I still think it would look worse than what you just did. I'm sure I'd projectile vomit. It would go on and on and I'd look really awful."

As our session ends I feel slightly deflated that in spite of my best efforts, Mary hasn't had a dramatic epiphany about her condition and then remonstrate with myself for being so naïve. I reflect on the fact that Mary's presentation is far more complex and long-standing than Jess's panic disorder and I will have to try harder.

Later that week I discuss the outcome with my clinical supervisor. He is impressed by my enthusiasm and amused by the small drama but suggests that perhaps my intervention was too premature. It would have been helpful to have done some preliminary work to loosen up Mary's belief in addition to the psych-oeducation. Why not focus on her childhood memory as it seems to be the root of the problem?

When we meet the following week, I explain to Mary that I want to conduct an experiment that will involve returning to her childhood memory of being sick during the Judo class. She does not have any objections so I ask her to relax in the chair, close her eyes, and go back to that time as if she were there now as her adult self. I have asked her to describe to me what is happening moment by moment as though I am blindfolded, relying on her description. Because the memory is so vivid, Mary has no difficulty in doing this.

"I'm walking through the entrance on the ground floor and up the narrow steps to the first floor where there's a reception desk. The first thing I am noticing is the smell. It's slightly musty, I think it may be the matting but there's also a slightly medicinal smell like disinfectant. I'm at the entrance of the training room now and I can see the girls practicing groundwork on the mats. It's very bright and the walls are all painted white. There are large mirrors along the front wall. I can see the instructor wandering between the girls advising them on what to do."

"Where is little Mary?"

"I can see her at the other end of the training hall by the changing area and the door to the shower. A bigger girl is grappling with her and little Mary is looking very unhappy, her face is very pale. The older girl has pulled her on top really violently and little Mary is grimacing. Suddenly she is sick over the older girl and they both stop. Everyone has stopped and they are all looking at little Mary. The older girl looks disgusted and some of the others have started laughing."

At this point, I can see a tear running down Mary's cheek so I ask her to pause the image. I invite her to approach little Mary, get down on her knees, and look into her eyes. I ask what she can see.

"She looks so scared and confused—she doesn't know what to do."

"What do you want to do to help her?"

"I'm wiping the sick off of her face with my handkerchief. She's crying now so I'm hugging her and telling her that it's ok and that she's done nothing wrong. I'm looking at the other girls and the instructor. They have all stopped laughing and they look ashamed."

I am using the Arnoud Arntz (Arntz and Weertman, 1999) protocol for imagery rescripting that we first encountered in Chapter 1 when I worked on Ross's childhood memories. According to the protocol, I would usually complete the first part of re-living the experience from the perspective of Mary's adult self and then begin the whole episode from the start again but from little Mary's perspective. However, Mary appears to be deeply immersed in the experience and is finding it intensely emotional so I don't want to risk breaking her state of concentration. I instruct her to become little Mary at that moment and ask her what she needs from older Mary.

"I am hugging older Mary tightly and I feel safe in her arms. I ask if she can clean me before we go home. She takes me into the shower and washes me with warm water. She helps me to dry myself and get changed. She puts the Judo suit in a bin in the changing room and we leave. She has her arm around my shoulder and I feel protected as I walk pass the instructor and the other girls. I ask her if she will come home with me and she tells me that she will always be there to protect me. We are on the street and the sun has come out, it's a nice day now. I feel clean and happy to be out in the open with Mary."

I am always amazed at the powerful effect this technique has on clients and how easily they are able to switch perspectives from their adult self to their younger self and back again. It's a moving experience to see someone rescuing their "inner child," and Mary has done a fine job. After Mary has re-oriented herself back into the therapy room, we sit in silence for a while. The session is nearly over and I feel it appropriate to let Mary leave without any discussion about her experience. My intuition tells me that her mind will be processing her new experience of the memory long after she has left the room and I don't want to disturb this delicate state.

When we meet the following week, Mary tells me that she has dreamt about the memory twice and on each occasion her older self-intervenes and cares for her. I ask her what she makes of this and she ponders for a while before replying.

"It was a really strange experience but somehow when I go back to that memory, I don't get the feeling of shame anymore. It feels as though they should have been ashamed, the instructor and the girls, about the way they behaved towards me. The other thing that's occurred to me is, what would my future self say to me now about the way that I'm wasting my life because of this fear. I tried to imagine having a conversation with my 45 year old self and she was telling me that I really need to break free of this."

"And do you have any thoughts on how you could achieve this Mary?"

"I've got to act now because if I don't seize this moment, I'm going to lose it and I'll be stuck for the rest of my life. I think I have to go into that supermarket across the road but I really have to do it right now."

I'm a little taken aback by the vehemence in Mary's determination and am slightly concerned about the weight of her expectations about this impetuous act. However, it may be the only opportunity to help her to face her fear and disconfirm her belief about how awful the outcome will be. It will be helpful if I can encourage her to make some sort of predication or she may learn nothing in spite of her leap of faith.

"If we go into the shop Mary, what's the worst thing that might happen?"

"I'll be sick and the people in the shop will be disgusted."

"On a scale of . . .. "

"Can we just do it please!" She is getting angry because she feels incredibly anxious and wants to get this over with. I fetch my jacket and we leave.

My anxiety increases as we approach the shop, and I notice that Mary is sipping water from her bottle; her face is ashen. The store is a humble minimarket rather than a supermarket and has three compact aisles. The floors are covered with slightly shabby lino, and at the moment we are the only people present apart from the shopkeeper who is stationed behind his till. I am watching Mary very closely and suddenly she pauses, makes a retching sound, and bends forward. Her shoulders start to shudder and her face contorts as her retching increases. She brings up a small amount of grey bile accompanied by strenuous heaving. The shopkeeper has left his till to see what's going on but doesn't intervene. Slowly Mary straightens herself, and I pass her a handful of tissues. She wipes her mouth and tears are streaming down her face. As we leave the premises, I momentarily consider apologising to the shopkeeper but dismiss the thought as it might confirm to Mary that she had committed a shameful act. I make a mental note to apologise later on during the day and offer to make amends in some way (a deposit in the charity box?). I congratulate Mary on her bravery but she seems downcast and doesn't speak to me as we return to the therapy room.

When we are seated, I ask her what she made of the experience. She dabs her eyes with a tissue and replies.

"I don't know what I expected but I feel disappointed, flat."

"I can understand that. You had really worked yourself up and the bravery it must have taken after all this time was incredible. It seems to me as though you expected some sort of break-through, a feeling of freedom or something similar?"

"I think your right, and it wasn't a big deal. It feels like an anti-climax." I am concerned that Mary's expectation of a huge epiphany is blinding her to the positive aspects of what has just taken place and try to gently encourage her to review the event from a different perspective. I take out my mobile phone and retrieve the formulation I had sketched out on the whiteboard a few weeks ago and hold it in front of her.

"Do you remember your prediction of what would happen if you were sick in public? You told me that you would 'projectile vomit'. What actually happened back there?"

"Not much."

"It looked to me as though you were struggling to be sick, am I right?"

"Yes, I thought to myself, I have to see this through, so I stayed there."

"So you could have left the shop if you wanted to. That tells me that you've got more control over your reactions than you've thought up until now. What do you think?"

"Yes, I suppose you are right."

"And what about your prediction that other people would judge you negatively?"

"The man in the shop didn't say anything."

"That's correct—a similar reaction to the people standing outside the bakery when I pretended to be sick the other week. The fact is, most people will think that you're ill if you're sick in public unless you look inebriated in some obvious way." I can see that I have managed to regain Mary's attention and although she does not display any overt enthusiasm, the feeling of despondency within the room had receded slightly. Noticing that our time is running out, I make one further attempt to encourage Mary before we end.

"You've made a fantastic breakthrough Mary, please don't lose that momentum. It's natural that you might feel a sense of anti-climax after you've expended so much nervous energy building yourself up for what you did. Please don't lose sight of what you've achieved and also what you've learned." Mary nods grudgingly.

"Where do we go from here?"

"Now it's all about reclaiming your life. What I'd like you to do before we meet next week is to write a list of all the situations you've been avoiding over the past year. The plan is to help you develop confidence by tackling each of these situations one step at a time. We'll start with the easier ones and work upwards."

And that is how our work continued for the remainder of our time together. Mary was able to gradually re-engage in all of the mundane but necessary routines of life that she had been avoiding due to her fear. She managed to visit shops, post offices, and banks again during the daytime rather than skulking around late at night. She also managed to drop her safety behaviours and managed to queue without sipping from a water bottle. But in spite of her apparent success, Mary actually became more depressed as our therapy was coming to an end and I felt quite despondent. I shared my feelings of disappointment with my supervisor as a way of coming to terms with what seemed to be a rather unsatisfactory ending to therapy. Our discussions helped me to see the inevitability of Mary's low mood following her therapeutic "breakthrough." For the past year, Mary's life had revolved around a mundane but predictable and safe routine. In spite of the frustration that had brought her into therapy, she didn't realise the price she would have to pay to achieve freedom from her cocooned life. Now there was no longer a reason not to re-engage with all of the challenges that life brings and the slow climb to re-integrate within society. Mary admitted to feelings of loss and regret for the past year during which time she had put her life on hold. But she also felt huge trepidation at the prospect of re-building her career and entering into new friendships, perhaps an intimate relationship. Instead of being excited at the prospect of reclaiming her life, Mary felt weighed down by the thought of how much effort it would take.

This sort of ambivalence is often described in the world of psychology as *secondary gain*: the client derives an advantage from their illness and is either consciously or subconsciously aware of this. Sigmund Freud (1917) originally coined the term and although it can be used in a dubious way (e.g. inferring malingering in someone suffering from a physical or psychological illness), clients often display this sort of conflicted thinking when they achieve success in therapy. I try to normalise this for Mary and she concedes that part of her wants to cling to the security of her sheltered existence but another part of her wants to battle on and make the most of her life. She acknowledges that her mood is low and that she spends a lot of time brooding about her life. The goal of getting into therapy had given her the hope that she would overcome her problems. Now that she has achieved what she set out to do in therapy, she realises that there is another steep hill she will have to climb and she feels exhausted at the prospect. I suggest that she might benefit from attending her local NHS CBT for depression group (named "Mood Management" as opposed to the less appealing "depression group") and she hesitates. The local NHS run various groups that are delivered by psychology graduates. Whilst they do not have the advantages of individual therapy in terms of tailoring the approach to fit the patient, the groups do not require a long wait and impart helpful knowledge that clients can put into practice immediately if their presentation is not too severe. I explain to Mary that there is another potential benefit for agreeing to this course of action. By taking part in a group, she will develop further confidence and carry through the momentum of our work together. She agreed with my suggestion with some reservations, and we agree that I will contact her in 3 months' time to see how she is getting on.

Three months have gone by very quickly and the note in my diary reminds me that it's time to call Mary to see how she is doing. She answers immediately and sounds reasonably cheerful. As the conversation goes on, it becomes apparent that Mary's life has not changed a great deal since our last meeting. She is more active during the day and hasn't relapsed in terms of avoiding situations due to her previous fear of vomiting. She now eats breakfast in the morning and is trying to give up smoking. But she hasn't engaged in any job-seeking activities and seems hesitant about taking this next step. I offer to put her in touch with the National Careers Service to provide support with this but she declines. I run through the clinical measures with her to verify whether her symptoms of anxiety and depression remain acceptably low and this proves to be the case. We agree that she no longer needs help from me and I conclude the call by reminding her that she can contact me at any time if the need arises. I feel slightly flat after the phone call and wonder whether the reason for this dip in my own mood is due to me imposing my own agenda on Mary. I consider that my own phantasies about what clinical recovery should look like may be different from Mary's revised ambitions. Perhaps she needs a period of consolidation to build up stamina before taking steps to rebuild her life and seek more challenging work. Or perhaps she is too exhausted at the prospect and prefers to stay within her comfort zone with her hard-won new freedoms. Unless she contacts me I'll never know as I don't want her to think that I'm hounding her. Sometimes the hardest part of the job is letting go when you remain uncertain as to whether or not your work has made a lasting difference in someone's life.

Caitlin's Story

My first impression of Caitlin is that she is very well-dressed, highly professional in her appearance, well-groomed but sitting awkwardly. I soon find out that the reason for her physical awkwardness is that she is wearing a nappy, one of her many safety behaviours to manage her constant anxiety about the possibility that she may soil herself. Like Mary, Caitlin has reconnoitred the area on the way to her first appointment with me and knows exactly where the toilets are in case of an "emergency." Caitlin explains that this is a recent development. She has been, she tells me, a worrier for as long as she can remember and a "bit of a perfectionist," but this latest problem has developed unexpectedly and now has a profoundly negative impact on her life.

The problem began the previous year when Caitlin suffered from a stomach virus that was not medically diagnosed but resulted in her suffering from chronic diarrhoea for 2 weeks. She said that after this event, her stomach "did not seem normal" and was constantly bloated. A couple of weeks later, she travelled to Kent by train to visit her mother and was constantly anxious in case she had to use the toilet on the train and potentially embarrass herself in public. Caitlin has always been concerned about the possibility of other people hearing her "make unseemly noises or smells" in the toilet, and this is consistent with her apparent perfectionism: she wouldn't like other people to think of her in the context of these humble but necessary bodily functions.

Shortly after her trip to Kent, Caitlin started working for an IT company based within her local area and she became obsessed with the consistency of her stools and the constant churning feeling in her stomach. She returned to her GP who took a sample of her faeces to check for stomach infections and inflammatory bowel disease or IBD. Once IBD had been ruled out, Caitlin's GP suggested that she may be suffering from irritable bowel syndrome or IBS and suggested that she may benefit from a course of CBT, hence her appointment with me. Caitlin is somewhat sceptical and slightly annoyed at the inference that this disturbingly physical problem is "in her head." I make a mental note to proceed carefully with any explanation around the psychological aspects of her condition and frame subsequent questions as delicately as I am able. She has clearly suffered a lot over the past year and, as she continues her narrative, it becomes apparent that IBS and her response to its symptoms have had a major impact on her life.

Fortunately, I had attended a one-day workshop the previous month delivered by a wonderful Professor of Psychology as Applied to Medicine from the Institute of Psychiatry by the name of Rona Moss-Morris. I got into a conversation with her during the break and said that she made IBS seem a compelling subject, I think she took this as a complement, and she was very passionate about her area of expertise having worked in it for years. We both agreed that the event organisers possessed a wry sense of humour as they had scheduled the workshop for 14th February – Valentine's Day. The knowledge that Professor Moss-Morris imparted on that day would prove invaluable throughout the course of my work with Caitlin.

Irritable bowel syndrome is described within the category of medically unexplained symptoms because it is often difficult to diagnose (Hunt, 2016). The main symptoms include:

- Abdominal pain and cramping
- Change in bowel habits
- Bloating and swelling
- Flatulence
- Urgent need to use the toilet

But these symptoms are also common to a number of other disorders. The Rome Foundation is a not-for-profit organisation conducting research into gastrointestinal disorders, and they have published helpful criteria for diagnosing IBS (Lacy et al., 2016):

Recurrent abdominal pain, on average, at least 1 day/week in the last 3 months, associated with two or more of the following criteria:

- *Related to defecation*
- *Associated with a change in frequency of stool*
- *Associated with a change in form (appearance) of stool.*

Criteria fulfilled for the last 3 months with symptom onset at least 6 months before diagnosis.

IBS is very common and affects 10–22% of the population. It affects twice as many women as men. It accounts for approximately 240,000 UK primary care consultations per year and costs over £200 million per year in NHS time. IBS affects the sufferer's social and occupational functioning—quality of life is significantly lower for IBS sufferers (Nellesen et al., 2013).

Interestingly, given Caitlin's comments about her perfectionistic tendencies, individuals with *negative perfectionism* are more likely to suffer from IBS (Moss-Morris, 2019). With this tendency, you need to constantly achieve high levels of performance to prevent "bad" things from happening in life as opposed to *positive perfectionism* which is helpful as it is motivational. With negative perfectionism, you just experience relief for achieving an outcome; positive perfectionists celebrate the outcome. This tendency is often present in top athletes.

There are recent hypotheses which consider that IBS and IBD may be linked to disruptions in the human microbiome and Emeran Mayer (Mayer, 2018), executive director of the UCLA Center for Neurobiology of Stress, has written about this topic in his book, *The Mind-Gut Connection*. We know that the *enteric nervous system* plays a major role in IBS. This is what gastroenterologists sometimes describe as "the brain in your gut" (Hunt, 2016)—the nervous system within the stomach that is responsible for *peristalsis:* helping to break food down with digestive juices ready for absorption. One theory of IBS is that motor neurons in the brain and the sensory neurons contained within the enteric nervous system may become *hypersensitive*. If you don't suffer from IBS or a similar condition, you're less aware of normal activity within your gut. But for sufferers of IBS, a gas bubble moving along the gut gets picked up by the sensory neurons and transmitted to the brain as an alarm signal. This is referred to as *visceral hypersensitivity:* being hypersensitive to any sensation within the viscera or gut. In addition, the action of food moving through the colon, or *motility,* can react negatively to certain types of food. When you add an anxiety response from the *sympathetic nervous system,* you have a vicious cycle between the brain and the gut. As in Caitlin's case, many people develop IBS following food poisoning or a similar illness leading to a temporary bout of chronic diarrhoea. Unfortunately, the memory of the event is often so aversive, that sufferers like Caitlin live in dread of a recurrence and visceral hypersensitivity sets them up to feel every sensation in their gut. And if an unexpected bowel movement and its social consequences are your biggest fear, you have a perfect storm.

Caitlin has developed a range of behaviours calculated to prevent her worse fears from coming true but unbeknownst to her, they have become part of the problem in maintaining her vicious cycle. She has started to engage in a number of safety behaviours including trying to empty her bowels before leaving home and taking Imodium in the morning, afternoon, and evening to prevent "accidents." These safety behaviours have become so extreme to the extent that she rents a flat very near her workplace so that she can dash to her toilet at short notice and she has taken to wearing nappies at work "just in case." As well as emptying her bowels before leaving home, Caitlin restricts eating, plans any route she takes for proximity to toilets. She immediately checks for the location of toilets in venues and now avoids all travel on public transport. Whenever she leaves her flat, Caitlin constantly scans her body for symptoms of loose bowels. I am surprised that Caitlin has been so candid in describing her symptoms and behaviours but she tells me that she doesn't mind talking to me about this as I am a "medical professional."

I have asked Caitlin to keep a daily record of her symptoms and behaviour as a starting point for our work together. This proves helpful as in our second session, Cailin has discerned from her diary that it's not accurate for her to say that she restricts eating, she only does this after she has left the flat. Before she leaves that flat, however, she engages in a very unhelpful process that she has recorded.

Caitlin discloses that he eats chocolate or what she describes as other junk food including crisps in the belief that it will induce a bowel movement before she leaves her flat ("If I eat crap, it will make me crap"). Her logic is that if she has a bowel movement before leaving her flat, she will be less at risk of experiencing an accident. Second, she eats large amounts of "junk food" and then goes to the toilet 10 to 20 minutes later. She gives the example of a 500 g bag of Mars bars. Also, once she has left her flat, she will avoid eating altogether to avoid the possibility of soiling herself in public. What she doesn't realise is that it can take 10 hours to several days for any food consumed to make its way to the colon (Everitt et al., 2015) rather than her 10- to 20-minute estimate and would account for some of the unexpected episodes at work that have sent her dashing back to the toilet in her flat. My immediate thought is to provide her with a mini-lecture based on what I know about IBS but resist the impulse.

The one thing that's constantly drilled into CBT therapists during their training and subsequent clinical supervision is to be more *Socratic* in their work with clients. Plato is credited with saying that the ancient Greek philosopher Socrates (c. 469–399 BC) was a man who thought for himself and taught others to think for themselves (Magee, 1987).

This endeavour is encouraged by therapists to facilitate *guided discovery*, using carefully targeted questions to help clients realise thinking errors and gain insights into how to overcome personal challenges. There are two schools of thought as to how you approach this task. In the first instance, neither you nor the client has the "answer" to their problem and you are working in collaboration through a method of question and answer. The other approach assumes that the therapist can see a possible solution that would help the client but guides them to this conclusion through questioning rather than just proving them with the answer. I find both approaches helpful depending on the level of self-insight and knowledge that the client has and right now I'm thinking that Caitlin would benefit from the latter method. I figure that the best starting point for both of us will be to map out the problem on the whiteboard in the same way that I had done with Mary. Based on what Caitlin had told me and following further questioning, this is what we come up with:

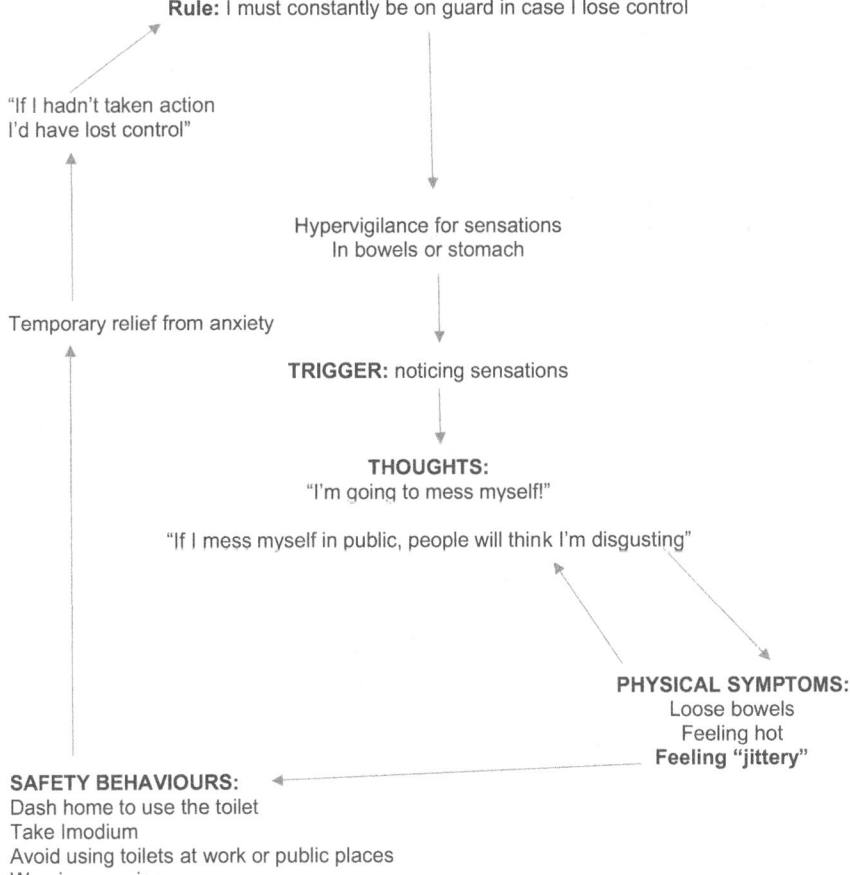

Rule: I must constantly be on guard in case I lose control

"If I hadn't taken action I'd have lost control"

Hypervigilance for sensations In bowels or stomach

Temporary relief from anxiety

TRIGGER: noticing sensations

THOUGHTS: "I'm going to mess myself!"

"If I mess myself in public, people will think I'm disgusting"

PHYSICAL SYMPTOMS: Loose bowels Feeling hot Feeling "jittery"

SAFETY BEHAVIOURS: Dash home to use the toilet Take Imodium Avoid using toilets at work or public places Wearing nappies

Figure 7.2 Formulation of Caitlin's Fear of Soiling

Caitlin stares at the whiteboard reflectively. She does not show any sign of an emotional reaction and asks various questions to clarify her thinking. She seems to be taking an analytical approach to her problem and is beginning to concede that there may well be a psychological component that needs to be addressed. We agree that I will contact Caitlin's GP to check what she has in mind with regard to treating the physical symptoms as Caitlin has mentioned a discussion around FODMAPS. Based on what I have read (Nanayakkara et al., 2016), carbohydrates called Fermentable Oligo-saccharides Di-saccharides Mono-saccharides and Polyols (FODMAPs) are thought to cause irritation to the bowels and may account for symptoms of IBS. Many GPs recommend a diet that eliminates sources of FODMAPS for 6–8 weeks. This covers a wide range of foodstuffs including fruit, vegetables, dairy, legumes, grains, and sweeteners. Following elimination, these high FODMAP foods are re-introduced individually to determine which of them trigger symptoms of IBS. I need to clarify that what I intend to put in place in terms of a treatment plan for Caitlin does not cut across anything the GP has in mind. In the meantime, I want to explore Caitlin's firmly held belief about how other people would react if she soiled herself—her deepest fear.

"What makes you think people would respond in that way Caitlin? From what you've said, this has never happened to you."

"Not as an adult but I remember once when I was at primary school I had an upset stomach and messed myself. A lot of the other children were horrible to me afterward and my parents had to move me to another school because I got so upset. I never want to feel like that again."

"Children can be very cruel sometimes but do you think that adults would act in the same way?"

"I think so, yes, I'm pretty convinced they would."

Similar to Mary's aversive childhood memory of being humiliated when she was sick over another child during her Judo class, Caitlin's early memory has been triggered by recent events and underpins her fear of how people would react to her if she were to soil herself in public. I continue to question Caitlin about her childhood and she tells me that after her parents transferred her to another school, she worked very hard to achieve academically but was quite withdrawn from the company of other children, something of a loner. Fortunately, the incident at the previous school did not result in a fear of soiling at that time, Caitlin did, however, report developing a certain fastidiousness about anything related to using the toilet. She would avoid using the school's lavatories at all costs other than to have a pee and also developed an aversion to using public lavatories. Her worse nightmare in adolescence and to the present day would be if someone overheard her making a noise whilst defecating or if they noticed a smell after she had used the toilet. At the same time, she developed a highly perfectionistic approach to her academic work that has persisted into her career, something Professor Jeffery Young (Young and Klosko, 1994) would describe as *unrelenting standards* in his work on *schema* or psychological "life traps." For Caitlin, this type of schema describes the belief that she can never be good enough in all that she does and that she must constantly try harder. Young maintains that individuals who hold these beliefs about themselves (without even knowing it) impose on themselves unrealistically high standards to avoid some inner criticism. Caitlin's perfectionism and attempts to control outcomes in life seem to be a way of overcompensating for the "imperfectionism" of her body and its fallibility.

Although Caitlin was sceptical about taking a psychological approach to her problem, she is increasingly willing to explore the possibility as the formulation makes sense to her analytical mind. She is also highly motivated to do something about the problem as it has prevented her from entering romantic relationships since her stomach virus the previous year and she confesses to feeling lonely. Once again, I am pondering on how to have the greatest impact in helping Caitlin with her problem. Her apparent lack of knowledge about her condition surprises me so I provide her with literature from Professor Moss and her colleagues' manual (BMJ Open, 2015) and ask her to provide me with a mini-lecture on IBS including the physiological and psychological aspects that contribute to the condition. She is happy with this "academic" task but I know that I need to make a start on addressing her negative belief about other people's reactions as soon as possible as my hunch is that if it remains unresolved, Caitlin will make little lasting progress. I have an additional task in mind and begin to sound her out.

"You mention that you work for an IT company. Have you ever carried out any internal staff surveys or taken part in them?"

"Yes, occasionally."

"This belief you have that members of the public would find someone disgusting if they had an "accident" in public. I wonder if there's a way we could test your 'theory' because at the moment we don't have any evidence for it."

"What are you suggesting, that I survey work colleagues? I spend all my time going to great lengths to conceal my problem and now you want me to draw attention to it?"

"Sorry, I didn't explain that very well. Not with work colleagues, but do you have a network of friends that you're in touch with—via Facebook for example?" I'm taking a bit of a chance at this point as I've never used Facebook and don't know a great deal about social media but am hoping that at 30 years of age Cailin is more tech-savvy than I am. To my relief, Caitlin confirms that she does and that in spite of being a loner at school, she has managed to make a number of friendships at university because this was a new environment and she had less fear of being judged. To my slight surprise, Caitlin agrees to carry out a survey with her friends asking what their response would be if they saw a professional-looking person (her words) soiling themselves in public. Cailin comes up with a subterfuge to draw attention away from herself by presenting the question to friends as part of a work-related survey. As I mentioned previously, I'm not a big fan of carrying out surveys to change clients' negative beliefs, but I thought it might be worth a try given that the target audience are Caitlin's friends and their responses may be credible to her.

When we meet the following week, Caitlin delivers a diligently prepared lecture on IBS, its causes, and maintaining factors. She is particularly fascinated by the workings of the digestive system, the role of the brain and the nervous system ("fight or flight" response) on the digestive process, and theories around the brain–gut connection. She now realises that her strategy of eating junk food to induce bowel movements before leaving the flat and restricting her diet exacerbate the problem, and she is now intent on increasing physical exercise, improving her diet and water consumption and has downloaded a mindfulness app to practice relaxation. This all seems too good to be true, and I ask Caitlin why she hasn't taken the simple step of researching her problem before now.

"I just didn't want to think about it anymore than I had to. It's been on my mind every waking hour and I thought that if I started going into even more detail, it would make the problem worse and I'd become even more obsessed."

Her response is consistent with that of many clients who become avoidant in confronting their problem, and in these instances self-help books are of limited use. I have experienced many occasions when clients have declined psycho-educational materials as homework during the early stages of therapy for fear that "it will make my depression/anxiety/OCD worse." Like Caitlin, gradually and with gentle encouragement, these clients eventually engage with an explanation of their condition that they had previously avoided, and this simple intervention can often enable them to make a dramatic breakthrough. Therapy provides them with a safe space in which to explore their condition, something that may have threatened to destabilise them had they attempted to do so by themselves.

Caitlin had not been able to carry out her survey, but in our next session she presents the results. She managed to survey 15 friends by asking them the following question:

"If you saw someone professional looking who had messed themselves in public, what would you do and/or what would you think?"

Caitlin was surprised by the responses she received that most of her friends would feel sympathy and assume that the person was unwell. None of them were condemnatory. Most of them confessed that they had been in this situation at least once in their life and many said that they would help the person or ask if they needed help. However, she was still sceptical about what the response would be amongst members of the general public who were complete strangers and possibly less compassionate than her friends. I started to experience a sinking feeling that Caitlin's treatment plan would need a behavioural experiment to disconfirm her negative belief. I explore this with her in a tentative manner because I am already thinking of the potential consequences for myself.

"So we've already figured out that you've got this belief, '*If I mess myself in public, people will think I'm disgusting*'. How strongly do you rate your belief on a scale of 0 to 100?"

"Before I did the survey, I would have said 90%. Now it's more like 75%."

"Great, I'm glad that was of some use. If you *didn't* have that belief, what effect would it have on the way that you act now, on all these safety behaviours and how you live your life?"

"Well I've learned that fear is a big factor in all of this and it's contributing to a vicious cycle between my gut and my brain. And I guess that if I didn't *care* what people might think if I had an accident, I'd be less vulnerable to getting triggered by physical symptoms of anxiety—I might be able to break the cycle, gradually I suppose."

"It might be a little unrealistic to aim at not caring what people think. Most people would be *concerned* if they had accident in public but they might not see it as a catastrophe. What would help prove to you that strangers wouldn't necessarily view you as disgusting if you had an accident in public?"

"I don't know. Maybe if I saw it happen and watched other people's reactions. But that's very unlikely to happen and there's no way I'd put myself in a situation where it might happen to me."

"What about if it happened to me?"

"What?"

"What if I pretended to soil myself in public and you watched other people's reactions?" Caitlin's response is disappointingly matter of fact. I had been quite nervous about putting myself forward for this particular experiment and was expecting a little astonishment after working myself up to my "grand reveal" but all I am rewarded with are sceptical questions that I find a little deflating.

"How would you do it and make it look realistic?"

"I would make it look very realistic—I have various methods."

"Ok, anyone could fake something visual but what about the smell?" I hadn't thought of making the experiment *that* realistic but realise that I have backed myself into a corner with this one.

"I could make that realistic too."

"Ok, I'm willing to try it. You're the expert and I guess you've done this kind of thing before." In the same way that Caitlin felt at ease talking about her symptoms of IBS with me, she now seems to think that I am comfortable with the prospect of pretending to soil myself in public because I am a "medical professional." Before we end the session, I obtain Caitlin's predictions on how the good people in the local neighbourhood will respond to my faecal antics:

Someone will say something negative 95%.

People will act visibly disgusted (pull a face) 95%.

People will look and laugh 90%.

People will stare and point 90%.

People will move away in disgust 90%.

The prospect of this particular behavioural experiment hangs over me like a dark cloud for the remainder of the week, and I realise that, in spite of some of the other challenging behavioural experiments I've carried out, I have always tried to maintain a modicum of dignity, even when pretending to vomit in a bin. The prospect of wandering up the high street with my trousers covered in fake shit and smelling evilly does not fill me with glee.

That evening I begin my preparations. Research on Google leads to me narrowing down the choices for one of my props for the experiment: "Waste Turd Prank Poop Joke Fun Novelty." A colleague who carried out a similar experiment told me that she had used chocolate mousse but I suspect that wouldn't look very convincing: onlookers would probably think I had sat on a Mars Bar. The next thing I turn my attention to is an olfactory prop—not something I can obtain on Amazon. I contact my daughter-in-law and ask if she will do me a small favour: could I please collect one of my youngest grandson's nappies, post-use? She works in an A&E department as a nurse and is not particularly squeamish and understands the clinical rationale behind my request. I collect my grandson's contribution to the experiment sealed in a nappy bag and drive home feeling confidence in the props but uncertain about the outcome as this is the first time I have tried something of this nature.

I meet Caitlin in a quiet side street the following day having prepared my props. The High Street is nearby and a constant resource for me in conducting behavioural experiments although this one doesn't feature that regularly. I apply the "Waste Turd Prank Poop" to the seat of the old denims I have chosen to wear for the occasion and Caitlin confirms that it looks "lumpy and realistic." I outline my plan. We will walk down the High Street together and pause near any stationary shoppers. I will feign physical discomfort and manoeuvre myself to present a view of my soiled derriere. At that moment, I will surreptitiously open the nappy bag concealed within a Sainsbury's plastic carrier. I provide Caitlin with an olfactory preview, and she wrinkles her nose although still seemingly nonplussed at my careful preparations.

As we walk onto the High Street, my anxiety starts to increase as it does on these occasions but a little more than usual. It's an early spring morning, and there is a happy bustle of activity in the clear sunshine after weeks of grim, rainy weather. Perhaps the local shoppers will be in good spirits and lenient towards my antics. We approach a bus stop where a few people are waiting, mostly elderly, and a mother with a child in a buggy. I totter about in front of them holding my stomach and wincing, positioning myself so that they can get a full view of my begrimed trousers seat. My hand trembles slightly as I reach into the plastic carrier, open the nappy bag, and begin what I hope is a discreet wafting action. No reaction at all. The small group ignore me and look into the distance for sight of a bus or look at the ground; an elderly lady steps back to adjust her position in the queue for my tottering movements. I lurch off to find another small gathering with Caitlin in tow and repeat the process drawing a similar lacklustre response. I reason to myself that at least I didn't provoke an outwardly hostile reaction and decide to return to the therapy room with Caitlin to deconstruct the whole episode.

I have changed out of my grubby denims, disposed of my grandson's nappy, and am sitting opposite Caitlin. I ask her what she made of our experiment.

"Nothing happened, nobody reacted." She looks bemused, even less impressed than Mary was at my vomiting experiment. I point to the whiteboard where I have noted Cailin's predictions from the previous week and observe that nothing of the sort happened. How would she rate her predictions now were she to have an "accident"?

"Well, they've probably come down a bit, I couldn't put a figure on it. But it's one thing to have an accident in front of a bunch of strangers on a high street and another if I were to mess myself in front of work colleagues. I'd be mortified and I still think their reaction would be negative."

After our session has concluded, I experience a tension headache as the adrenaline begins to subside and I feel dejected. As I reflect on what happened I recall something that Professor Adrian Wells said about setting up behavioural experiments for panic attacks (there are similarities between this and fear of soiling). He maintains that the experiment needs to induce physical sensations that are a close match with the feared symptoms (Wells, 2008). This principle applied to the hyperventilation provocation experiment I carried out with Jess in Chapter 6 where encouraging her to over-breath induced the same feelings of dizziness that she experienced when having a panic attack and proved that she could not faint when her anxiety and blood pressure were high. In this instance, the experiment that I set up for Caitlin did not closely resemble the *circumstances* of her feared catastrophe: soiling herself at work in front of colleagues who knew her rather than strangers in a high street. I would have to admit defeat and concede that this time I would not be able to set up a suitable experiment in spite of my stressful and messy attempt this morning.

At our next session, I resort to a less dramatic approach and we construct an exposure hierarchy for Caitlin to work on:

Exposure	Anxiety Rating
Using the toilet at work	85
Travelling to Kent without Taking Imodium	80
Leaving home without going to the toilet	70
Travelling to central London without taking Imodium or wearing a nappy	75
Attending work without taking Imodium	60
Attending work without wearing a nappy	50
Eating lunch at work	40

Over the next few weeks, Caitlin makes steady progress and manages to reduce many of the safety behaviours that she had clung to desperately over the past year. She has found that making basic changes in her lifestyle, such as improved diet, exercise, and meditation, is yielding unexpected positive results. She is also working with her GP on the FODMAPS diet and is hopeful that if she is able to identify and eliminate problem foods, she will be able to reduce her symptoms of IBS or make a full recovery.

Two sessions before we are due to end our work together, Caitlin informs me that she has started dating again. She tells me that she met her new boyfriend online and started facetiming one another. They were both mutually attracted to one another and the early candour that developed between them gave Caitlin the courage to disclose the challenges that she had experienced over the past year. I expressed delight at this positive development as Caitlin had expressed feelings of loneliness when she started therapy. I automatically assumed that she was maintaining an online relationship with her new boyfriend but she surprised me by intimating that he had stayed the whole weekend at her flat "without incident."

"John was totally unphased when I told him about my little problem. He told me early on that he used to do voluntary work in an old peoples' home and was used to many "accidents" although I did rather resent the suggestion that he could clean up after me as though I was in my dotage."

Caitlin is smiling at this thought, and I am beginning to think that her new boyfriend is rendering my role superfluous. It seems that his evident affection for Caitlin and down-to-earth view of human physical functioning is having a therapeutic effect, and she seems far more relaxed about the idiosyncrasies of her body, far less perfectionistic.

When we reach our final session and part company, Caitlin is well on the way to recovery and I remind myself that often in CBT, success comes from facilitating a process devised by experts rather than introducing dramatic experiments. I recall attending lectures delivered by Glen Waller, an expert in eating disorders and Professor of clinical psychology at the University of Sheffield. Glen has written and lectured on the concept of *therapist drift* (Waller, 2009) and the dangers of straying from evidence-based CBT protocols due to the clinician's notions of creativity and my experience with Caitlin is a sobering reminder. Nevertheless, I still find the notion of *fidelity with flexibility* a helpful guiding principle (Sanetti, Collier-Meek and Fallon, 2016).

References

American Psychiatric Association. (2013). *Diagnostic and statistical manual of mental disorders*, 5th ed. Washington: American Psychiatric Publishing.

Arntz, A. and Weertman, A (1999). Treatment of childhood memories: Theory and practice. *Behaviour Research and Therapy*, 37, pp. 715–740.

Boschen, M.J. (2007). Reconceptualising emetophobia: A cognitive-behavioural formulation and research agenda. *Journal of Anxiety Disorders*, 21, pp. 407–419.

Davidson, A.L., Boyle, C. and Lauchlan, F. (2008). Scared to lose control? General and health locus of control in females with a phobia of vomiting. *Journal of Clinical Psychology*, 64(1), pp. 30–39. Published online in Wiley InterScience.

Everitt, H., Landau, S., McCrone, P., Bishop, F., Little, P., Chalder, T., Moss-Morris, R. and BMJ Open. (2015). Regular 8: A self-management programme for IBS, manual for ACTIB trial, 5, p. e008622. doi: 10.1136/bmjopen-2015–008622

Freud, S. (1917). *Introductory lectures on psychoanalysis*. London: Hogarth Press, Vol. 16, pp. 378–391, 1959.

Hunt, M.G. (2016). *Reclaim your life from IBS*. New York: Sterling.

Lacy, B.E., et al. (2016). Bowel disorders. *Gastroenterology*, 150, pp. 1393–1407; Rome III Diagnostic Criteria for Functional Gastrointestinal Disorders.

Magee, B. (1987). *The great philosophers*. London: BBC Books.

Mayer, E. (2018). *The mind-gut connection*. New York: Harper Collins Publishers.

Moss-Morris, R. (2019). *CBT for irritable bowel syndrome workshop delivered 14th February 2019*. London: Institute of Psychiatry, Kings College London.

Nanayakkara, W.S. Skidmore, P.M., O'Brian, L., Wilkinson, T.J. and Gearry, R.B. (2016). Efficacy of the low FODMAP diet for treating irritable bowel syndrome: the evidence to date. *Clinical and Experimental Gastroenterology*, 9 (June 17), pp. 131–142. doi: 10.2147/CEG.S86798. eCollection 2016

Nellesen, D., et al. (2013). *Journal of Managed Care Pharmacy*, 19(9), pp. 755–764.

Sanetti, L., Collier-Meek, M.A. and Fallon, L. (2016). Fidelity with flexibility: Treatment acceptability and individualized adaptations of evidence-supported treatments. doi: 10.1093/oxfordhb/9780199739134.0.013.25

Veale, D. (2009). Cognitive behaviour therapy for a specific phobia of vomiting. *The Cognitive Behaviour Therapist*, pp. 1–17. British Association for Behavioural and Cognitive Psychotherapies.

Veale, D. and Lambrou, C. (2006). The psychopathology of vomit phobia. *Behavioural and Cognitive Psychotherapy*, 34, pp. 139–150.

Waller, G. (2009). Evidence-based treatment and therapist drift. *Behaviour Research and Therapy*, 47, pp. 119–127.

Wells, A. (2008). *Cognitive therapy of anxiety disorders—a practice manual and conceptual guide*. Chichester: Wiley.

Young, J.E. and Klosko, J.S. (1994). *Reinventing your life*. New York: PLUME. Published by the Penguin Group.

Chapter 8

And COVID

When the first lockdown was announced on 23 March 2020, the situation presented psychological therapy services with a profound challenge: how do you provide a therapy that has traditionally required two people to sit in a room together for 50 minutes having a meaningful discussion? Even CBT, which can be very task-oriented, requires the therapist to pay close attention to the patient's tone of voice and body language sometimes evaluating micro-expressions. The answer was similar to that of many occupations. The work had to continue and therapists needed to adapt their practices and become more adept at videoconferencing technologies.

During the first few weeks of lockdown, there was an intense flurry of activity with therapists striving to become proficient with the new technologies and undergoing a paradigm shift: adapting their clinical practice to ensure that clients still received high-quality interventions that emulated the intimacy of the clinic room but delivered remotely via videoconferencing. This endeavour was supported by various centres of excellence such as The *Oxford* Centre for Anxiety Disorders and Trauma (OxCADAT) who very quickly adapted CBT protocols for remote access working and circulated the materials and guidance to clinicians free of charge. This was phenomenally helpful as one of the immediate challenges facing therapists was dealing with the constraints of delivering a form of therapy that often relies on carrying out behavioural experiments with or without the therapist outside of the clinic similar to the examples described in previous chapters. How, for example, do you cure someone of social anxiety such as Martin who we met in Chapter 5 without exposing them to social situations? OxCADAT (2020a) suggested a range of imaginative adaptations such as arranging group conversations with two strangers on webcam and giving a presentation to a virtual audience. A particularly helpful recommendation for adapting trauma therapy was the use of Google Maps to support clients being treated for PTSD in making virtual site visits (OxCADAT, 2020b). This procedure is often carried out towards the end of therapy as a form of exposure once the client's symptoms of PTSD (e.g. nightmares and flashbacks) have been treated, and they are encouraged to visit the location where the traumatic event took place. The purpose of the visit is to help the client to overcome fear associated with the location, and it often leads to a

DOI: 10.4324/9781003091745-9

powerful sense in the individual feeling that they have reclaimed their life after months or perhaps years of suffering. I was initially sceptical about this method and doubted that it would generate anything like the emotional intensity of a real site visit. However, after a great deal of practice I used the Google Maps site visit with a client who had been involved in a horrific terrorist incident and he vouched for the intensity of the experience finding it demanding but therapeutically effective at the same time. Accompanying him on the virtual site visit and having intimate knowledge of his experience felt surprisingly immersive.

In addition to getting to grips with new technology and adapting clinical practices, therapists also had to adjust to the emotional demands of remote working. Clients who were feeling emotionally vulnerable due to their original psychological challenges were confronted with the added burdens of isolation and increased uncertainty—both of these huge factors in increasing symptoms of depression and anxiety. Reported suicidal risk increased nationally and with it the need for clinicians to manage this risk whilst working from home.

Although mechanisms to support therapists were still in place from the outset of the lockdown including clinical supervision and training, many therapists reported the emotional burden of working in a home environment with traumatised clients appearing on screen and for some young therapists this meant being trapped in their bedroom within a house share. Many clinicians reported missing working in a therapeutic setting during the early restrictive phase of the lockdown when it was only permissible to leave home for 1 hour of exercise each day. I missed the ritual of commuting to and from the clinic and the ability to maintain clear boundaries between work and home. It was often difficult to experience the constant emotional residue hanging over your personal living space following a suicidal risk management exchange or a particularly disturbing therapy session such as listening to clients recount memories of childhood abuse. Turning to a colleague at the clinic after these encounters offered a rapid means of debriefing and processing the emotional aftermath. I found it difficult to pick up the phone and call colleagues for the same purpose—it felt as though I would be intruding into their busy work schedule.

I noticed the quality of my sleep deteriorating over this period and experienced frequent bouts of insomnia. This was probably not helped by a huge increase in coffee consumption to sharpen my mental focus during hours of therapy delivered via videoconferencing. When you are in a therapy room it's far easier to inject energy into the session when the client's reserves are flagging perhaps by getting up and using the whiteboard to illustrate a learning point or collaborate on working through a particular problem. Far more difficult to do this via a computer screen in spite of interactive features or, for many clients, just a mobile phone screen, I found myself working twice as hard with facial expression, gestures, and tone of voice especially with clients suffering from depression.

In spite of these challenges, therapists adapted their practices and continued to support their clients. But it soon became apparent that for some clients remote access to therapy would not be possible. This included, for example, clients who had a disability that would render therapy via telephone or videoconferencing impossible. Likewise, clients who were in danger of domestic abuse in their home. This required a different approach and involved working with these clients face-to-face but there were certain requirements therapists had to adhere to including wearing face masks during sessions which provided an added challenge during therapy when so much is conveyed through facial expression.

One of the clients that I treated during this period reminded me that although delivering therapy under these circumstances was challenging, other frontline workers had to cope with far harsher challenges, such as Consuela. She and her husband were supermarket delivery drivers and had come to England from Spain several years ago to find work. She enjoyed her job and diligently served the local community until one day 6 months ago when a young man racially abused her during a road-rage incident when he threw a brick through her cab window. Consuela had suffered from nightmares and flashbacks following this event. When I picked her up for treatment, she disclosed that she had suffered the double misfortune of a near-death experience having been admitted to hospital suffering from COVID. She was now presenting with symptoms of PTSD arising from her experiences of COVID and we agreed to target this memory in treatment. Consuela had researched various forms of treatment for PTSD and had specified a preference for EMDR or to give the treatment its full name, Eye Movement Desensitization and Reprocessing. Along with CBT, I am fully trained and accredited in EMDR and was able to help Consuela.

Before I share Consuela's story of recovery with you, I'd like to tell you something about EMDR as, in my experience, it is a remarkable form of therapy and has a fascinating history. EMDR evolved due to a random observation by its originator, Francine Shapiro (2018), latterly Senior Research Fellow Emeritus at the Mental Research Institute in Palo Alto, California who sadly died in 2019. According to Francine's own account of events, she was out walking one day in the spring of 1987 when she paid attention to a series of disturbing thoughts that had occurred to her, but more importantly, she noticed the way they had suddenly dissipated. Francine observed that disturbing thoughts have a repetitive quality to them and play over and over in the mind and this is certainly common in rumination, a mental behaviour we encountered in Chapter 2 that maintains depression. Francine eventually noticed that when she experienced the disturbing thoughts her eyes moved back and forth in a rapid upward diagonal motion until the thoughts disappeared. She was surprised by this effect and deliberately recalled the disturbing thoughts. To her further surprise, the thoughts had reduced their emotional impact. This led her to deliberately bring to mind disturbing thoughts and memories whilst practicing the same eye movements all with the same ameliorative effect. Intrigued by what she had stumbled upon, Francine approached colleagues and friends and asked them if they wanted to work on "nonpathological" psychological issues. They volunteered disturbing memories and present-day frustrations that they were experiencing. Francine asked them to emulate the way she had moved her eyes back and forth but discovered that most of her subjects were unable to maintain the same muscle control to continue with the eye movements she had shown them. She then asked them to follow her fingers in the same direction and with the same tempo that she had used on herself and found that they were able to do this. They also reported feeling better about the memories following rapid eye movements. This led Francine to carry out her first controlled study in 1987 with rape victims, molestation victims, and Vietnam veterans who met DSM-III criteria (DSM-III; American Psychiatric Association, 1980) for a diagnosis of PTSD. Since Francine's random discovery in 1987, EMDR is now recognised as best practice for the treatment of PTSD in healthcare associations around the world including the UK National Institute for Health and Care Excellence (NICE) and the World Health Organization.

Incredible as the results are from using EMDR as a psychological therapy, it is still not fully understood how these amazing results are achieved but there are a number of theories. One of Francine Shapiro's earliest hypotheses (Shapiro, 1989) was that the rapid eye movements employed in EMDR trigger the same neurological processes that take place during REM whilst we sleep. Dr. Robert Stickgold (Stickgold et al., 2001; Stickgold, 2002) from the Harvard Laboratory of Neurophysiology suggested the same hypothesis that eye movements and other forms of stimulation used in EMDR such as tapping trigger physiological responses that lead to the reorganisation of memory in the brain—similar to memory processing that takes place during sleep and, specifically, dreaming. During treatment, clients initially focus on a particularly disturbing aspect of their trauma memory but very often rapidly access other associated memories from the past or fragments of the trauma memory that they had forgotten. For example, a client I had treated who had been physically attacked in a public place suddenly recalled the memory of being comforted by a passer-by. This aspect of the memory had remained hidden from the client for 2 years since her experience of the trauma and its recollection helped her gain a different perspective of the event: although she had been attacked, she realised that there were people who are prepared to help and were kind to her.

EMDR offers other advantages when helping clients to process traumatic memories. As we have seen in previous case studies, shame is often associated with memories of childhood sexual abuse and it can be extremely challenging for the client to talk about the event. In these instances, the clinician can use a *blind therapist protocol* in which the client focuses on an aspect of the trauma memory without describing it whilst experiencing the eye movements. In my experience, clients often disclose the memory after a few sessions as their feelings of shame have dissipated due to the reprocessing. This occurred when a client described a particular aspect of a memory that she had not wished to describe to me at the start of treatment: being arrested and led out of her home in handcuffs. This had come about because her husband and business partner had committed fraud and embezzlement. She was subsequently released, and her husband went to prison and, in spite of her innocence, the feelings of shame associated with the arrest were seared into the client's memory long after she had been exonerated.

You may be wondering, how can you use EMDR with a client who is blind or otherwise visually impaired? The treatment has evolved to meet this challenge and includes alternative *bilateral stimulation* methods including administering alternate taps to each of the client's hands or asking them to listen to alternating tones. The theory is that getting the client to focus externally on the stimulus (e.g. tapping) whilst they experience the internal distress of the trauma memory will activate brain functions that enable processing to take place. Shapiro noted that these alternative methods to eye movements have been used since 1990 and have been clinically effective (Shapiro, 1994). I have used these methods many times including my work with a client who had lost one eye falling from a ladder (his trauma memory).

Although eye movements or alternative bilateral stimulation form a major part of EMDR treatment, there are other important aspects. An important preparatory phase involves the use of calm or safe place imagery. This typically involves getting the client to recall a pleasant and calming event. Popular choices are holiday memories but in some instances, clients who have experienced particularly traumatic pasts are unable to recall any memories of feeling safe. In these instances, it's necessary to help them to create an imaginary "safe place." Fortunately, Consuela is immediately able to bring to mind a memory of walking with her husband in the Alhambra, a Moorish fortress in Granada, Southern Spain. She described walking through palace gardens and beautiful patios whilst surveying the distant Sierra Nevada Mountains. In order to help her become totally immersed in the experience, I encourage Consuela to imagine the event unfolding moment-by-moment in real time and ask her to pay particular attention to her senses. I ask her to describe what she can see, hear, feel, smell, and even taste. She closes her eyes and describes her experience to me. I also close my eyes and am transported to Al Andalusia with her.

"I am walking through a sun-lit patio surrounded by thin columns with horseshoe arches. In the centre of the patio is a circular fountain supported by marble lions; jets of water pour out of their mouths and catch the sunlight. I pass through the columns into a large chamber with high ceilings and look down into a green courtyard with carefully sculpted hedges and tall Cyprus trees, their fragrances rise up to me. I walk out onto an open terrace and I have a panoramic view of Granada, its magnificent white buildings towering over the Darro River and behind the city the peaks of the Sierra Nevada mountains under a bright blue sky."

I ask Consuela how she feels as she is walking through the palace and she tells me that she is completely at peace and happy. I ask her where she feels this and she smiles, gently placing her hand on her heart. I reluctantly asked her to gradually bring her attention back to our therapy setting and notice the feeling of the chair she is sitting in before opening her eyes. At moments like this, I'm often prompted by a selfish urge to prolong this particular exercise to gain respite from the hectic routine of the day as well as for the benefit of the client.

After Consuela has reorientated herself, I complete the procedure by asking her to think of a word that vividly evokes the memory she has just revisited. Without hesitation she says "Alhambra," the name of the palace she walked through. I tell her that this is her "access" word. Whenever she is feeling stressed she can recite "Alhambra" and recall the feeling of calm associated with the memory. We test the efficacy of this technique as I want to be confident that Consuela will have the ability to self-soothe at will if she experiences any trauma symptoms such as flashbacks or nightmares between our sessions. I have explained to Consuela that during the early stages of EMDR therapy it is quite common for clients to experience an increase in these symptoms as the brain continues to process the trauma memories long after the session has finished. In order to test her ability to calm herself, I ask Consuela to bring to mind a recent incident when she felt mildly distressed. She recalls having an argument with her partner in a supermarket 2 days ago about which cat food to buy—apparently her partner's previous economy-priced choice led to the cat suffering from a bout of diarrhoea and a protracted cleaning-up operation in their flat. Consuela dutifully brings up the memory and describes feelings of annoyance and hurt when recalling the angry exchange. I encourage her to use her access word and she reports back that the unpleasant emotions associated with the memory have melted away and she is momentarily transported back to the serene and fragrant environs of the Moorish palace.

Having established a calm place that Consuela can retreat to for respite, we turn our attention to her primary trauma memory and I follow a very specific procedure to prepare the way for our work together. Consuela becomes very tense as she recalls her memory of being in a COVID ward in hospital surrounded by medical staff wearing face masks. I ask her to tell me what image or picture represents the worst part of the memory.

"It is Nurse Jenny holding my hand. It was at the point when I was about to give up and they would have put me on the ventilator. I knew that if they did that, I would have given up completely, I would have died."

I make a note of Consuela's description and ask her what negative thoughts she has about herself now in relation to the memory. She tells me that she still feels unsafe even though she is making a good recovery.

"When you bring up that part of the memory and those words, 'I'm not safe', what emotions do you feel right now?"

"Fear, real fear."

"And on a scale of 0–10 where 0 is no disturbance or neutral and 10 is the highest disturbance you've ever felt, how disturbing does that part of the memory feel now?"

"10"

Finally, I ask Consuela how she would prefer to think about herself in relation to the memory

"I am safe now—I fought COVID and won."

I ask her how the words feel to her on a scale of 1–7 where 1 feels completely false and 7 feels completely true. She settles on 4 which gives me cause for optimism as I've had many clients who give a rating of 1 at this stage.

At this point, I get up and arrange our chairs so that I am sitting diagonally opposite Consuela. The position is sometimes described as "ships that pass in the night," and it will enable me to pass my right hand from side to side in a horizontal motion whilst Consuela tracks the movement of my fingers. I ask her to guide me as to the proximity of the eye movement and whether she prefers to follow one finger or two—she opts for two. She tells me that she is comfortably able to track the eye movements and I ask her if she is ready to begin. She nods with a look of resignation. Before I go any further, I explain to Consuela that if she finds the experience overwhelming, she simply has to raise her hand and I will stop. She appears baffled by this instruction and I explain further.

"If you say "stop" during the processing I'll carry on because it may be something you said at the time of the event. If you raise your hand I'll take it as a clear indication that you want me to stop. Having said that, it would be better if you keep going even if it feels emotionally demanding because constantly stopping will prolong the experience and I want to help you get to the other end."

Consuela nods and I ready myself.

"Ok Consuela, I'm going to start the processing now. I'll guide you with what to focus on and I just want you to notice whatever comes up for you as we do the eye movements—just be curious. You might notice different thoughts, feelings or sensations in your body and other memories may occur to you. Or you might not notice anything other than the eye movements. There's no right or wrong reaction, it's different for everyone. Just notice whatever comes up for you and report it to me briefly each time I stop the eye movements. What I need you to do now is bring up the image of Nurse Jenny holding your hand at the moment you were about to give up and that thought, 'I'm not safe'. Now notice what you feel in your body right now and follow my fingers."

I begin the eye movements, and Consuela tracks the motion of my fingers from left to right. The recommended number of backward and forward motions within a set is 22 although EMDR therapists are advised to intuit this rather than count as the process would run the risk of becoming mechanistic. During these moments, the therapist endeavours to discern any indication of emotional change in the client. These cues can be overt, such as sudden tears or changes in facial expression. Or they can be more subtle, such as an increase in breathing or micro-expressions. Sensitive to these cues, the therapist often makes a decision to interrupt the set and ask the client what they notice. Getting the timing right is vitally important: if you intervene at the correct moment you will hopefully settle upon an insight or important shift in perspective that has entered that client's field of awareness during processing;

if you miss the cue and continue the eye movements, the client's internal narrative may move on beyond the point of insight. There is little subtlety about Consuela's response: her face grimaces and she shakes her head from side-to-side. I pause the eye movements, invite her to take a calming breath, and tell me what she notices.

"I just see darkness, death—I know I'm going there."

She is visibly shaking, and tears are running down her face.

"I don't want to do this thing."

We pause and I wait until Consuela has calmed down and taken a sip of water. I encourage her by saying that she has made a good start but I am considering that beginning with the most disturbing aspect of the memory may be too overwhelming for her. I consider my options and recall that my EMDR supervisor had previously suggested a grounding technique referred to as "circle of protectors" to enable clients to stay within the *window of affect* when they confront disturbing memories. This means getting the client to tolerate sufficient emotional intensity to facilitate processing the traumatic memories without becoming so overwhelmed that they dissociate or refuse to continue. This is achieved by enabling the client to feel as though they are partially back in the memory but partially in the room with the therapist and therefore safe despite the intense feelings they are experiencing. I begin to explore this approach with Consuela.

"I can see that you're finding this really challenging Consuela and I want to try to make it easier for you. The intense emotions that you're feeling are a really positive sign that you're beginning to process the memory but I want to help you to keep those feelings within a range you can tolerate. Can you think of someone whose presence comforts you, makes you feel safe?"

"Yes, my uncle. I used to visit him and my aunt in Madrid when I was a small child. I remember when they took me to Retiro Park and I got scared when I saw the Fountain of the Fallen Angel. He picked me up and hugged me and told me not to be afraid."

"Can you imagine that he's here with you now and he has his arm around you?"

Consuela's eyes moisten and she nods. I ask her where she feels this sensation of safety in her body and she places her hand on her chest indicating her heart. I ask her to focus on the feeling of her uncle comforting her and get her to track several slow eye movements. I ask her if she can think of anyone else who gives her this sense of protection and she suggests her mother. I ask her to imagine her mother and uncle placing a protective arm around her and notice what this feels like. Again, I get her to track another set of slow eye movements and she reports feeling soothed. We continue in this fashion until she has assembled her circle of protectors consisting of her uncle, mother, aunt, and a childhood friend. I am intrigued that she does not include her husband as she speaks of him with fondness but decide not to pry. I ask Consuela if she feels able to return to the memory of Nurse Jenny holding her hand at the point when she was about to give up but this time with her circle of protectors around her. She consents and we begin again. This time she is able to continue with the eye movements and when I finish the set and ask her what she notices, she tells me that Nurse Jenny is telling her to fight. She says with passion:

"I know that I'm a fighter!"

Throughout each session, the narrative of Consuela's trauma memory becomes more elaborate and she gains insights that were previously concealed from her: the kindness of the medical staff who cared for her and remembered acts of her own bravery and dignity in the face of fear and mounting despair. During our fifth session, she is suddenly able to get past the memory of being trapped in the COVID ward about to be put on a ventilator. We start with the most disturbing aspect of the memory and as the processing gains momentum, the words pour out of her as she tracks my fingers. This is what she described over the course of the session each time we paused between sets of eye movements.

"I can feel the mask on my face, the pressure, pushing down, I feel this terrible tiredness. The nurse is wearing PPE equipment, I can't see her eyes. I know it's her hand holding mine but all I can feel is a rubbery glove. Its making a squeaking sound as if the glove doesn't fit properly. **Consuela is crying now.** I can hear her Jamaican accent and she's telling me that I've got to be strong but I'm saying in my head, I can't be strong, I can't go on. I can feel the tightness in my throat. I'm telling myself, I've got to be strong but I'm scared. I can see the beds opposite—the people—the masks. They're permanently in their masks lying in the beds—I don't want to be like them. I've got to get out now!

It's like a tightness all around me **She begins coughing violently.** My breathing, my throat, my back.

Nurse Jenny is telling me to fight for my life. I know that if I give up, they'll put me on a ventilator and I won't come back from that. I want to get through the door and go back to the sea, I have to get back to the sea in Spain. I want the light, not the dark. The dark is a scary black place that's forever, the light is going home to Spain. The feeling of wanting to go home hurts down my face and neck. There is a battle going on in my head, I want to go home. I'm battling with the darkness, I'm trying to come out of the dark. I'm taking deeper breaths—it's hard but I'm fighting. I need to pull myself back from the darkness. The light is the good place to go, not the darkness. I have an image of home and Carlos and our cat.

I can see the oxygen gauge, I can see that it's in the middle. I know it's improving and it's giving me hope. I notice everything is becoming clearer, the light is coming on. I know the room is dark but everything feels lighter. I know that I've made it—I don't want to do it again.

I fought back and didn't give up hope. I wouldn't use a commode, I went to the toilet.

The door frame looks like it's getting nearer. I'm looking at the curtains in the light and I'm on a different ward—the good ward before I'm going home. I can feel the excitement, the impatience of waiting for my wheelchair to go home. The porter appears with the wheelchair—I'm going home! The feeling of tightness in my back has gone and I feel lifted. I'm hugging my bag, making sure I have everything. I'm going home to see Carlos and my cat, it feels amazing **Consuela is laughing.** I can see Carlos at the door and I know how close I came to dying, it's overwhelming **Consuela is in tears again.** And now Carlos is hugging me but I realise that I haven't seen him in two weeks—he is crying and I know that he really must love me! I know I've done it, I feel relief. I notice the lightness outside the hospital, I feel very small going out into a big space, going outside into the light."

During our eighth session, I check how disturbing Consuela finds the memory of Nurse Jenny holding her hand at the point when she was about to give up and she rates her level of disturbance at 0. When I ask her why this has decreased so dramatically, she tells me that when she looks back on the memory, she realises that she would never have given up because she is a fighter. That desperate moment of doubt in herself that was seared into her memory has been updated with the positive insight that the EMDR processing had facilitated. Her belief in the statement, "I am safe now—I fought and won" was 7: full conviction.

Over the course of the next four sessions, Consuela was able to successfully process the memory of being racially abused during the road-rage incident recalling positive memories of a female customer who invited Consuela into her home and comforted her after the incident whilst she was waiting for the police to arrive. We both attributed this rapid processing of the memory to the success she had achieved with the more challenging COVID ward memory. I think that we had both found it an intense experience in our own ways as I was surprised to find myself waking up several times during our weeks of working on the memory following a recurrent dream of being suffocated. I can only think that images from Consuela's memory played into my worst fears about contracting COVID during that period of heightened anxiety.

After we parted company, I made contact with Consuela a few weeks later as she had told me that she intended to visit the hospital where she had been admitted and the focus of our work together. I was curious to know how she would get on and was delighted with her report on the visit.

"I managed to visit the Hospital where I was treated for COVID and I didn't feel anxious at all. I spoke to one of the doctors who was part of the team that saved me, it felt wonderful, I was so grateful to them all. He told me that my lungs were over three quarters full at the time and I realised how lucky I was to have survived. The doctor told me that my lungs are now only a quarter full and he's really pleased with my progress. I'm still signed off work and before I return, Carlos and I are going to take a short holiday. We're going to stay with my cousin in Malaga and we're going to the sea. It's what kept me going in hospital and I don't care about the weather—I'm going swim in the sea even if it's raining."

References

American Psychiatric Association. (1980). *Diagnostic and statistical manual of mental disorders*, 3rd ed. Washington, DC: American Psychiatric Association.

OxCADAT. (2020a). *Cognitive therapy for PTSD (CT-PTSD): Guidance for conducting memory work remotely*. Oxford, England: Oxford University Press.

OxCADAT. (2020b). *Oxford Centre for anxiety disorders and trauma cognitive therapy for social anxiety disorder (CT-SAD): Guidance for conducting treatment remotely during the coronavirus pandemic* (Version 1). Oxford, England: Oxford University Press.

Shapiro, F. (1989). Efficacy of the eye movement desensitization procedure in the treatment of traumatic memories. *Journal of Traumatic Stress Studies*, 2, pp. 199–223.

Shapiro, F. (1994). Alternative stimuli in the use of EMD(R). *Journal of Behaviour Therapy and Experimental Psychiatry*, 25, p. 89.

Shapiro, F. (2018). *Eye movement desensitization and reprocessing (EMDR) therapy*, 3rd ed. New York: Basic Principles, Protocols and Procedures and The Guilford Press.

Stickgold, R. (2002). EMDR: A putative neurobiological mechanism of action. *Journal of Clinical Psychology*, 58, pp. 61–75.

Stickgold, R., Hobson, J.A., et al. (2001). 'Sleep, learning, and dreams": Off-line memory reprocessing'. *Science*, pp. 1052–1057.

Acknowledgements

My journey as a CBT therapist within the NHS would never have got started without the opportunity provided to me by the IAPT service's clinical lead at the time who took a chance on me just before Christmas in 2009. It was a particularly severe winter's day when I made my way to the interview, and heavy snow had caused chaos on public transport. I literally had to walk from Bromley to the hospital in west London apart from taking a couple of trams that were still running for a few stops having got up in the early hours of the morning to get there for my 9.30 am interview. It transpired that a number of interviewees had failed to turn up due to the adverse weather conditions so luck was with me on the day narrowing the odds of a successful outcome. Amazingly, further confidence was placed in me 2 years later when I was promoted to the role of Senior CBT therapist and the service lead for long-term health conditions.

I am eternally grateful to the clinical lead and my other supervisors for the wisdom that they have imparted over many years and also to the IAPT senior management team that I have worked with.

I'd like to make special mention of all IAPT therapists and pay tribute to their phenomenal hard work, dedication, and compassion as they regularly go the extra mile for their clients.

I'm grateful to all of my supervisees for making clinical supervision such a stimulating if sometimes challenging process and from my perspective, our sessions have been a shared learning journey.

My deepest gratitude to all the clients I have worked with. I hope this book gives some indication of the courage and tenacity you have shown in striving to overcome your personal challenges in therapy—it's been a privilege working with you and you've taught me so much.

This book would not have come to fruition without the faith placed in me by Joanne Forshaw and Grace McDonnell, my publishers at Routledge Mental Health, who also showed great kindness by extending the manuscript deadline when my mother passed away whilst I was writing this book.

Thanks also to my friend Nick Velissarides for his enthusiasm, support, and helpful suggestions.

And finally, I have to express everlasting gratitude to my wife Stella who has continued to encourage me throughout my career as a CBT therapist and during the writing of this book, particularly during my most challenging moments.

Index

Note: Page numbers in *italics* indicate a figure on the corresponding page.